The Practice of Medicine in Three Continents

An Autobiography

by Abbas Sedaghat MD FRCP FACP

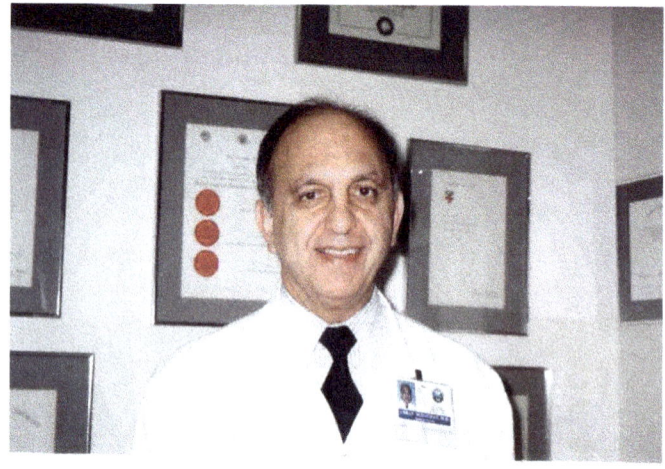

The author is a physician born in Iran, trained in multiple specialities in the United Kingdom and the USA, practiced in these countries as well as the Shiraz Medical Center in Iran.

Dr. Sedaghat is a Fellow of the Royal College of Physicians of Great Britain and became certified in Internal Medicine and Geriatrics in the USA, where he is a Fellow of the American College of Physicians.

He has a special interest and love for the teaching of clinical medicine to medical students and house officers. His love of teaching has won him multiple teaching awards at medical centers in three continents.

He is the author of several publications in prestigious medical journals. He lives in San Diego, California and has three children.

"Life is short and the art long, opportunity is fleeting, judgment difficult and experience dangerous. The physician must do the right thing at the right time."

- 1st Aphorism of Hippocrates

Chapter 1

School Days

~

"Please sir, can I have some more?"

I was about five years of age, some 75 years ago, when, during a stroll along Pahlavi Avenue in Tehran with my esteemed father, we came across a large mechanized vehicle with a red star painted on its side. My father remarked that the world was involved in a disastrous war and the large steel-clad machine was a Russian tank, and that Iran, the country of our birth, was in utter chaos.

It was on that day that he told me of his plans to send the family to the United Kingdom to be educated and to return to the country of our birth to be of service to the nation.

He also suggested that I should study hard and attempt to become a physician. Several years later, when I was nine years of age, we started our preparations to emigrate. A major factor that precipitated our move to Europe was the tragic death of our beloved mother because of severe postpartum hemorrhage during the birth of Sadegh, the third boy of the family, presumably due to the lack of facilities such as blood transfusion, I.V. oxytocin, and emergency hysterectomy.

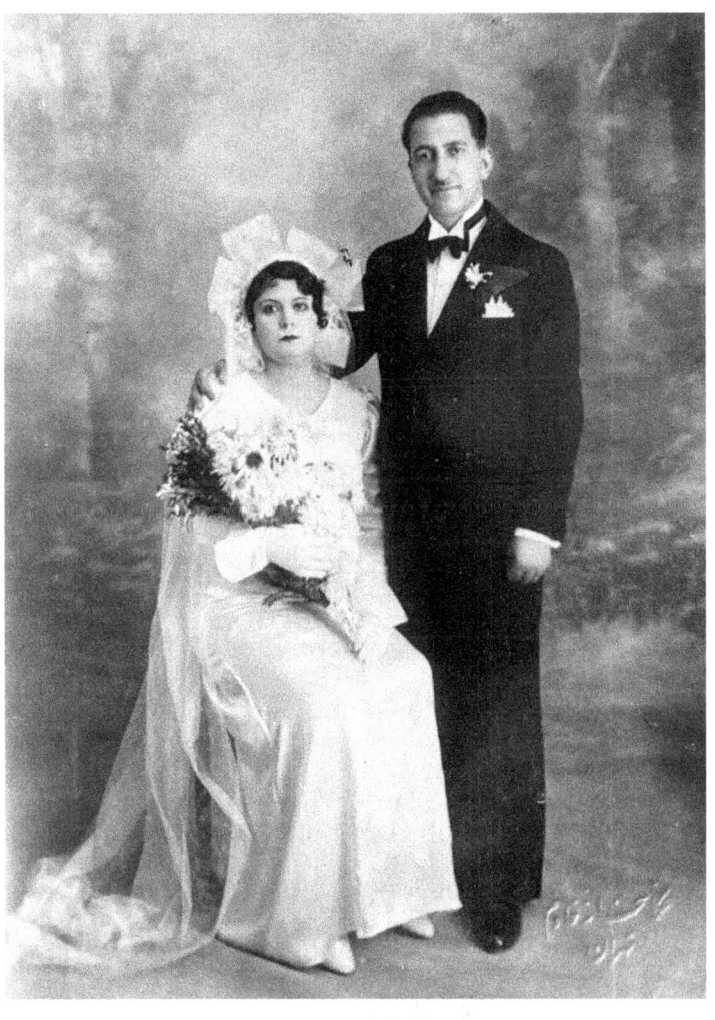

My parents at the time of their wedding in Iran.

Iran is an oil-rich country with most of the oil and gas found in the southwestern part of the country called Khuzestan. The Allies, requiring oil for continuing the Second World War, went ahead and removed for their purposes considerable amounts of oil and gas from this area. At this time, a member of the Parliament Dr. Mossadegh objected to the ready availability and use of Iran's natural resources for the war effort giving little or nothing back to Iran. He pleaded with the United Nations using this argument, but the Allies continued their illegal actions. Dr. Mossadegh, in a speech to Parliament, decided to nationalize the oil industry. This action resulted in the appearance of the British Fleet in the Persian Gulf.

Into the arena of this dispute came Dr. Mossadegh's frequent episodes of feigned loss of consciousness when things were not going his way. He would collapse frequently during sessions of the UN and a hospital bed had to be moved into the Iranian section of the UN for Dr. Mossadegh's frequent use.

My father worked hard and conscientiously for the benefit of the family. His father was a builder and built four housing units in Tehran just off Pahlavi Avenue, one for each of his four children. My father's work ethic resulted in his ability to build a house of substantial size in Shemiran, north of Tehran. There was a large and pretty garden surrounding the three-story residence. The Alborz range of mountains were easily visible to the north and Tehran, the large congested city, was to the south of our residence.

The house had several bathrooms, but a nonfunctioning boiler interfered with our regular use of the facilities. So to get cleaned up, we would make an appointment with the owner of a public bath, just south of our garden, get undressed in the sauna area of a private unit, get hot water poured over us, and a male person would arrive to give us a good rubdown and complete the job with a thorough soap and water combination.

On one occasion, he told me that the family was in financial difficulties when he was attending middle school. He decided to help the family by going to work at the Azarmi Pharmacy in Pahlavi Square. He kept up with his education by borrowing a friend's school notebook, going into the street and studying under the streetlight what he had missed in school that day. He would walk to the Azarmi Pharmacy during the winter's melting snow, in shoes that needed repair. Water would seep into the shoes freezing his toes. He was inquisitive and learnt a lot about medicines at the pharmacy. He went to Paris, France, later on in life to get his pharmacy degree.

He set up his pharmacy in Pahlavi Square, opposite the Azarmi Pharmacy. The front of the pharmacy was all glass with glass doors on each side. Customers were plentiful and would sit on comfortable chairs along each side of the waiting room. They would take their prescriptions to the reception table, behind which stood my father, who would provide them with their medicines made up in the back of the establishment where several mortars and pestles were in use.

He had an assistant, a Mr. Taee Khan, who was with him for many years. He was an honest and hard worker who would go to other pharmacies to get the prescribed medicine if it was not available in the Sedaghat Pharmacy. He would take the family kids to the Meehan Cinema to see Iranian and Indian movies, after which we would demand and receive cream puffs made at the pastry shop next door to the pharmacy before going home to sleep.

My grandfather (my father's dad) retired to the Holy City of Karbela in Iraq. I remember visiting him with my father in a rickety twin-engined aeroplane used for postal delivery. The plane was not pressurized and had to fly low. Through the windows and narrow spaces in between the metal plates forming the shell of the plane, I could see the people, their homes, the bazaars, and the domes of multiple mosques.

On Friday afternoons, the family gathered in our garden and festivities began. My cousin Manouchehr played the accordion accompanied by Mr. Tanha, the husband of one of my cousins who was an accomplished percussionist. Our grandfather, my mother's dad, was a renowned painter and visited us on Friday afternoons and brought with him paper and pencils, and tried hard to improve our drawing and painting skills. There was a chasm between my father's side of the family and my mother's. It wasn't too difficult to realize this divide. Even my aunt Zari, who was the family go-between, was silent about this issue.

When I was nine years of age, preparations were started to emigrate to Europe. The house was sold including all our belongings and we set off for Europe with SAS (Scandinavian Air Service). We were accompanied with our Aunt Zari, a very kind and selfless lady who had her own family and who were left to fend for themselves. The SAS flight made several stops for refueling during which time we recovered from our airsickness.

Our arrival in Paris was most welcome after the arduous journey, and because of fatigue and our unfamiliarity with the area in the vicinity of the air terminal, we ended up in a magnificent hotel nearby. It was palatial and reminded us of one of the Shah's palaces in Tehran. Because of the immense hotel costs, we decided to move to a more affordable apartment near the Tomb of the Unknown Soldier, a couple of streets away from the Avenue des Champs-Elysées.

There were several reasons why we stopped off in Paris on our way to the United Kingdom. The first was that the British authorities refused to issue a passport to our newly born brother saying that the war had caused a shortage of dairy products. The other reason was because our father had studied pharmacy in Paris several years earlier, spoke French fluently, and wanted to show us some of the sites of the beautiful city of Paris. It was rather fun for the youngsters in "Gay Paris." Sadegh had to be left in a foster home in the Paris suburbs and the excitement of being in Paris came to a sudden halt when the family proceeded to the county of the West Riding of Yorkshire in the north of England several weeks later.

We arrived with trepidation at the Old Swan Inn, situated in Gargrave. This was a pub with room for travelers on the way to Skipton and Malham. The Old Swan Inn pub was quite large and well attended by the locals. We spent several days preparing our uniforms and other school paraphernalia in the upstairs bedrooms. Gargrave was just a mile from Eshton Hall School, where the boarding school was situated.

Some five miles away was the market town of Skipton. This town had a castle, a church, and a wide central thoroughfare. It had a railway station with connections to various parts of northern England and Scotland. The town had two cinemas; near the cinemas was a large and busy bus station. To get to Eshton Hall School from Skipton, there was a bus that took one on to Gargrave, where one dismounted and walked through magnificent scenery of fields and hills covered by flowers and green grass being munched by cattle and sheep. There was a huge hill called Sharphaw some two miles from the school.

With much anxiety, the family made its way to the school. Communication was difficult because our knowledge of English was at best minimal. The headmaster and teachers were kind and understanding, but the indigenous boys and girls (Eshton was a co-educational institution) eyed the newcomers with some suspicion and disdain. We put up with the discomfort as best as we could and began the hard process of learning the ways of the English.

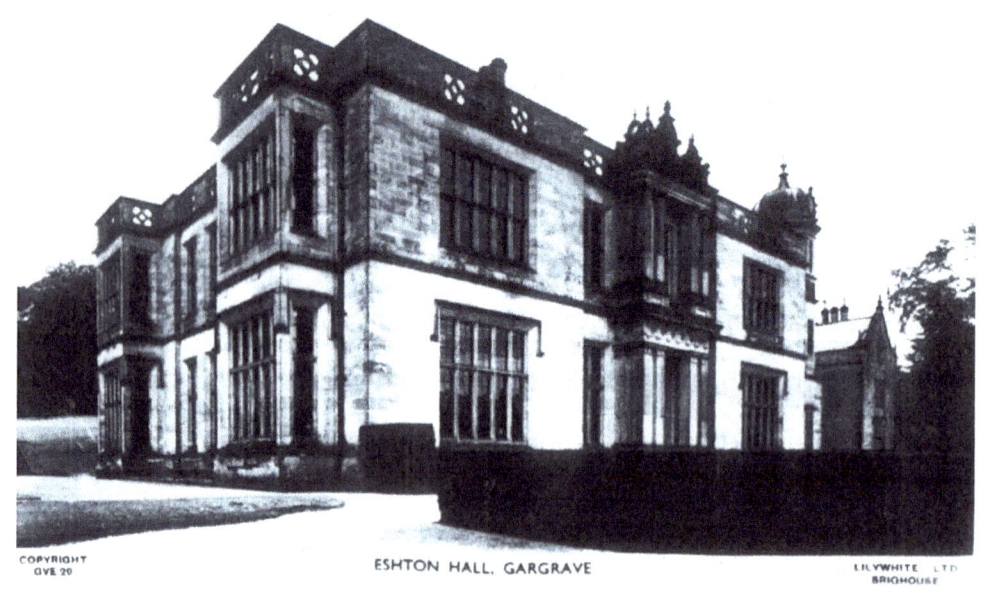

Eshton Hall School on our arrival in 1950.

The Headmaster welcomed us and showed us around the magnificent Eshton Hall, pointing out the gymnasium, science lab, the first to the sixth form rooms, the games room, the quiet room, the boys' and girls' dormitories, the teachers' room, and the large dining room. The presence of a relatively large foreign student contingent (from Pakistan, East Africa, and the Far East) was reassuring as was the presence of several students from Iran. All the same, we felt totally out of place, dejected, and lonely. My sister Gohar, my brother Reza, and I would seek each other out at break time (11:15-11:30am) and huddled next to the warm radiators (it was the winter term at the time) cried together in unison and at the bell, 11:30am, had to rush back to class.

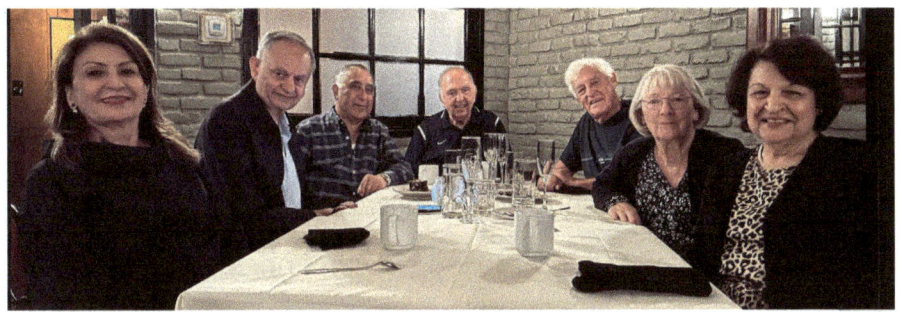

Some of the boys at Eshton School some 70 years later at a reunion in San Diego. From left to right: Banou, Razak, Farooque, Abbas, Jim, June, Farida.

Breakfast was at 8 am, lunch at 1 pm, and the last meal of the day was at 5 pm. A sizable handbell was on a table outside the tuck shop. The prefect of the day had to ring this bell at the times indicated above. The pupils lined up in single file along the corridor and each was closely inspected by the duty prefect before being allowed into the dining room. The areas inspected included their hands, shoes, and in some cases, the neck and the back of the ears for excessive dirt. Any deficiency had to be corrected before the pupil was allowed into the dining room.

The food was fairly nutritious but dispensed in smallish quantities. A staple was bread and margarine, served on each table, with water to drink. In the morning, there was cereal and milk; for lunch there was always mashed potatoes, carrots, beans and other vegetables, and occasionally, we'd get a piece of meat. Worthy of mention was the disgusting weekly offering of porridge, which I refused to touch. Several pupils demanded "more" as in the classic novel *Oliver Twist* by Charles Dickens, where the poor and hungry orphans came to the front of the dining room and pleaded, "Please sir, can I have some more?" This request was usually ignored and the hungry pupils had to seek out those who had access to the basement area next to the dining room, where large trunks filled with a variety of foodstuffs awaited the hungry owner. These trunks were prepared by the parents of a lucky few pupils and were generally filled with chocolate bars, tins of cookies, fruit like apples and oranges, and crisps (chips). The hungry pupils would wait around until the lucky students emerged from the basement with delicious snacks in their pockets and say, "Give us a bit mate." If the pupil was feeling generous, he'd share some; otherwise, he'd say, "Fuck off," and they were left hungry.

Within a couple of years, we had adapted to our new way of life and began standing our ground and giving as good as we got. Reza and I were soon instructed on how to tackle an opponent on the rugby field! I started in the first form aged ten and proceeded up the ladder to the fifth form participating in the school activities without any remarkable events. In the second form, the teacher Ms. Wright arranged for us to study our English Literature books, which kept our heads down and our eyes focused, whilst the Headmaster (Mr. Ron Purdy) came in frequently and chatted quietly with Ms. Wright. The latter was a pretty blonde single and seemed pleased with the attention bestowed upon her by the Headmaster.

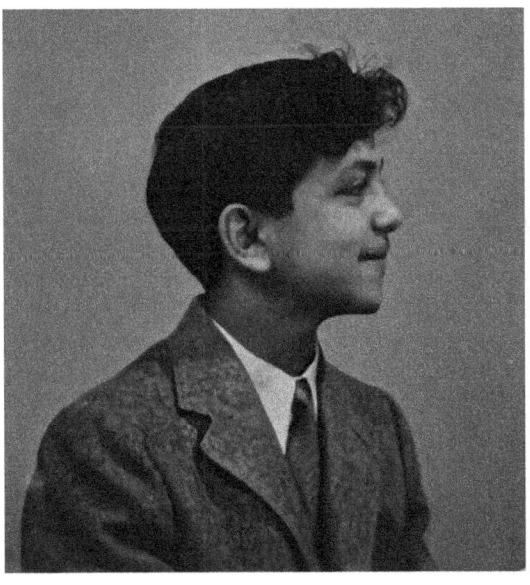

Abbas Sedaghat at age 12.

Every Christmas term, a choir was chosen, which performed in front of the whole school. My sister Gohar and my brother Reza were chosen as part of the choir. Mr. Hicks, who played the piano for the choir, felt that I was not good enough as a choir singer and thus I was excluded from the choir group.

A Mrs. Lee was the elocution teacher at Eshton. She stayed for 2-3 days every week and taught students the proper way to speak English. She was an accomplished actress in her younger days and was able to recite the whole of Shakespeare without any difficulty. Her favorite plays were *Hamlet, Julius Caesar, Henry the Fifth, Richard the Third*, and *The Merchant of Venice.* Those who did well were rewarded with one or more "pear drop" candies.

Unfortunately, Mrs. Lee passed away following a cerebral hemorrhage whilst at home at Scotforth House, Lancaster in the County of Lancashire in the mid 1960s. Mrs. Lee's residence named Scotforth House was quite gigantic. Many of the foreign boys and girls who had no home to go to during the holidays such as the Sedaghat's were taken in by Mrs. Lee.

A long time resident of Scotforth House called Mr. Cumstey (known by all as Skipper) took over the care of foreign students during the holidays following the passing of Mrs. Lee. He was injured in a car accident during the blackout of the Second

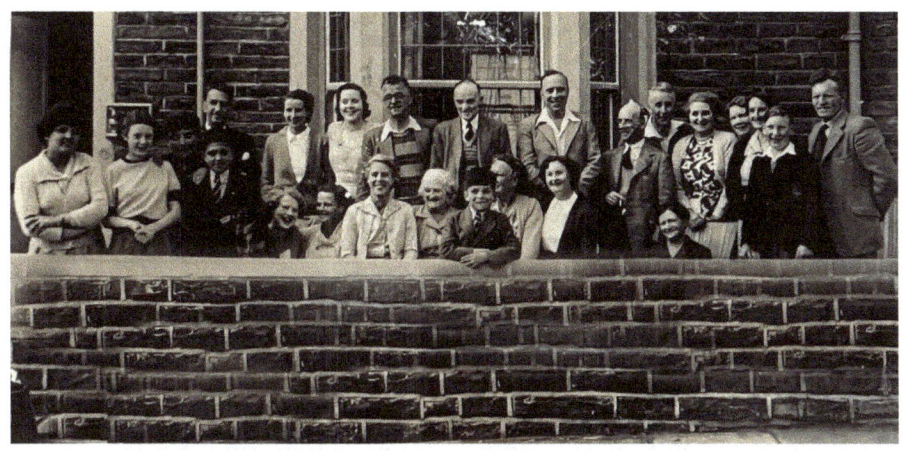

A holiday photo by the sea in Morecambe in the County of Lancasher. Gohar is on the far left, my father and I are third from the left, and Reza is in the middle of the front row.

World War. He sat at the top of the table during mealtimes. The food was good in quality and quantity and prepared by Ethel and her kitchen helper Christine. Skipper was the proud owner of a Daimler Benz car, which was large enough to accommodate all the residents of Scotforth House to be taken to a variety of professional competitions, including boxing, cricket, and rugby matches.

Once back at Eshton Hall School, talking back to a prefect resulted in my being caned by the Headmaster. The process consisted of bending over to touch one's toes and being hit on the bottom by specially made long wooden sticks. Those who had repeated beatings wore several pairs of shorts to decrease the pain and the resulting bruise marks! At this point, I should point out that I had a girlfriend, a pretty blonde girl, the same age as I, whose name was Pat Lodge. We often walked along the extensive areas around the school holding hands.

On one occasion, my brother Reza and I decided to go for a walk along the Woodland Path. This path was about a mile long and could be reached by crossing the river bridge at the bottom of the hill on which Eshton Hall School stood. The path was bordered by gorgeous rhododendron bushes and was used by those participating in the infamous marathon races.

Reza and I strolling along the path had to get out of the way of a tractor coming towards us. I stayed on the path, but my brother stepped aside between two rhododendron bushes and onto a bee's nest! All hell broke loose, and in a fraction of a second, bees were all over him, stinging him to their heart's content! The poor boy didn't know which way to run. Fortunately, the driver of the tractor came to our aid and using several rags, swatted away as many bees as he could from Reza. We hurried to the school clinic, where Matron dabbed every sting site with a pink-colored antiseptic cream. When she was finished with him, Reza looked like a circus clown wearing a red-spotted costume!

Bedtime was at 7:15 pm for the junior school and 8:15 pm for the seniors. Each pupil was provided with a bed, mattress, two sheets, a pillow, and a blanket. The winters were bitterly cold. As luck would have it, I often ended up in a bed next to the windows. These had to be open at all times, and I recall being covered in snow whenever there was a snow storm! In addition to the scant covering, the duty prefect inspected each pupil to make sure no socks, underpants, or vest (t-shirt) was worn under the pajamas. Such behavior was meant to toughen up the students!

My father paid the school a substantial amount for the children to go riding. A little way behind the school stood a building called the "lodge." On the ground floor were the stables where three horses were kept – Meg, Silver, and Brownie. The first two were gentle horses but Brownie loved to gallop when going along a grassy field. On one occasion with me on Brownie, he took off in a gallop with me terrified and hanging on to his neck for dear life. The horse stopped suddenly in front of a stone wall, and I flew over his head and crash landed on the soft grass without any significant injuries. My brother Reza started to cry every time he was put on a horse's saddle. He stopped his attempt at horseback riding quicker than expected. The horses were looked after by a Mr. Bateman, who used Brownie, ridden by a smallish Pakistani boy whose name was Khan, to participate in races at Skipton. They were winners in several races which made him and Mr. Bateman proud.

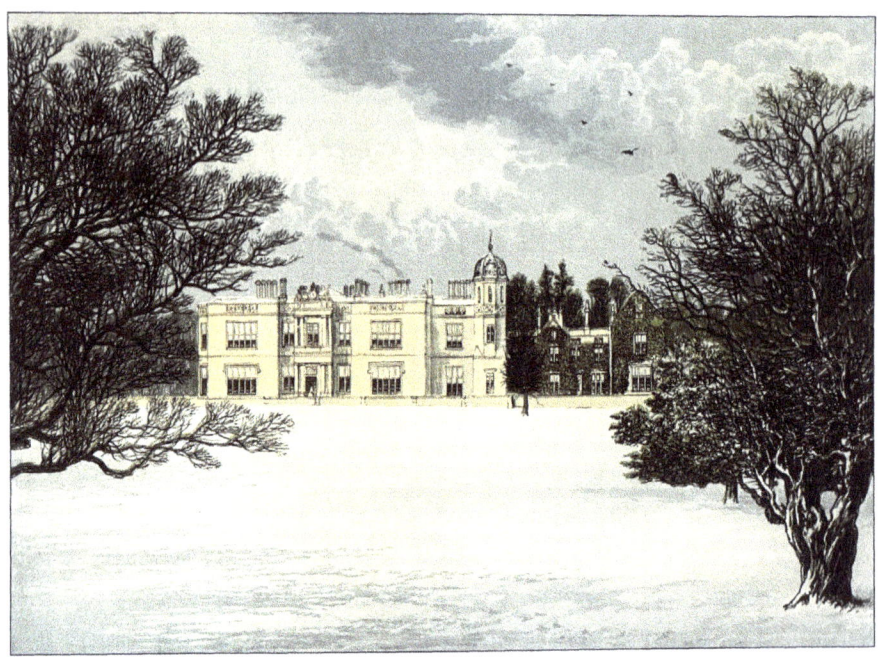

Eshton School during winter.

At Eshton Hall School, all boys over the age of ten years were automatically enlisted in the Army Cadet Force (ACF). Wednesday afternoons from 2 - 4pm was ACF time. Mr. Slee ran the show as well as being the school's art teacher, physical education instructor as well as filling in for any absent staff members. His rank in the ACF was Captain (three pips on each shoulder). The ACF at Eshton School was attached to the Duke of Wellington's Regiment stationed at the city of York. This Regiment played a major role in the British army in the Napoleonic Wars in Europe (1803 - 1815).

The enlisted members of Eshton School's ACF began as privates and were promoted to the rank of Lance Corporal (one stripe on each upper arm), Corporal (two stripes on each upper arm), Sergeant (three stripes on each upper arm), Staff Sergeant (a crown on each arm just above the three stripes), Sergeant Major, indicated by a larger crown over the wrists on both arms (as in my case), and promotion to an officer, as in Jim Mayor's case, followed by Captain, as in Mr. Slee's rank.

Eshton's ACF activities included getting on parade in a large area in front of the school with steps leading to the quiet room, marching smartly up and down the parade ground, practicing saluting on the march whenever we passed by Captain Slee, halting in unison, doing right and left turns on the parade ground, and about-turns whilst marching and from the standing position. Map reading was encouraged and target practice using 0.22 rifles and ammunition was a very popular activity.

The ACF went camping for 7 - 10 days every summer, joining other cadets from multiple parts of the UK. I recall a visit to Belfast in northern Ireland in 1958, where our unit won the rifle drill competition.

Exams, General Certificate of Education at the O (Ordinary) and A (Advanced) levels came and went without incident except that I had to attend the sixth form at Skipton's girl's high school to study biology, botany, and zoology, as there was no teacher at Eshton who could teach me these subjects. I went to the high school once a week for a period of two years, and it was embarrassing for me to be stared at by curious young ladies studying at that school.

This embarrassment was nothing compared to being forced by my father and his second wife (a member of the Naficy family), to haggle with British salespersons when purchasing goods at stores such as Harrods and other upscale shops in the West End. Haggling is a common practice in Iran, but in London the salespersons considered this behavior unseemly!

At this stage, I had been chosen to become Head Boy, Regimental Sergeant Major in the Army Cadet Force, Head of Lancaster House, and Captain of the School Rugby team. I should point out here that Eshton was quite a small school, and we often played against larger schools with good players, which meant that we often lost to our opponents. These so-called achievements resulted in my acceptance by St. Mary's Hospital Medical School in Paddington, London, to study medicine for a four-year period (1960-1964). This school of medicine, which was one of several other medical schools in London, was well known for the discovery of Penicillin by Sir Alexander Fleming for which he was awarded the Nobel Prize in Physiology and Medicine in 1945 and its reputation in fielding its rugby team, which provided several international players.

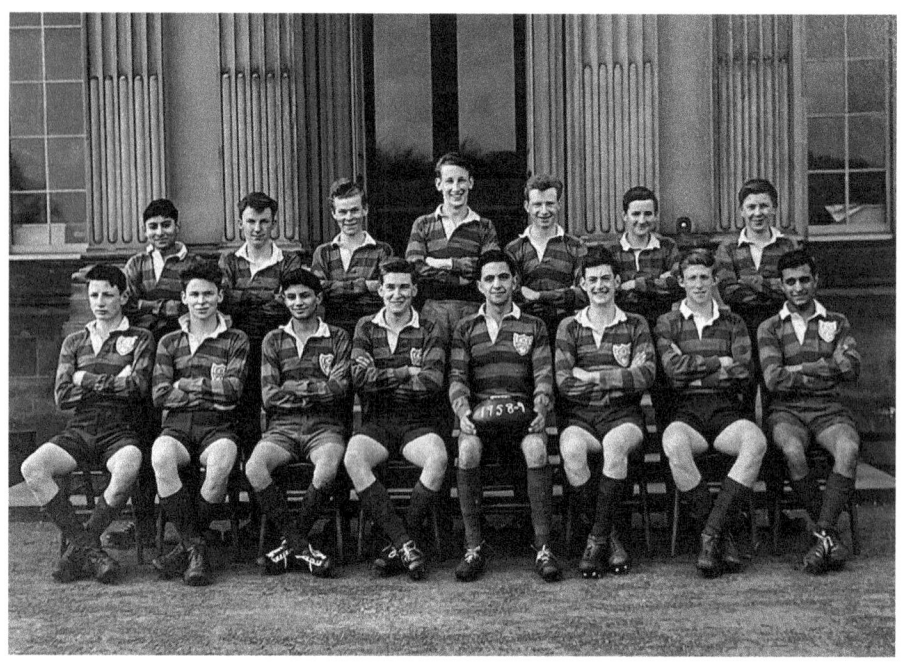

Eshton School's first fifteen rugby team in 1950. I am holding the ball in the front row. To my right is Anthony Knaggs who succumbed to acute Leukemia at an early age (the disease is now curable). To his right is Razak Dawood (who became the Finance Minister of the Pakistani Government in the early 2020s). Rafique Dawood is on the far left in the back row. Nanji (now a physician in Canada) is on the far right in the front row and second from the right in the back row is Jeremy Rowan-Robinson, the Headmaster's second son who became a Professor of Law in Scotland.

Chapter 2

He's a Mary's Man

~

"Where Penicillin was Discovered"

During my first year as a medical student, I shared a room with my friend and colleague James Nevill Mayor at a boarding house, efficiently ran by Mrs. Moxon a short distance from St. Mary's Hospital. Mrs. Moxon fed us well, kept our rooms clean, and made sure we were up at 7 every morning to be on time for the first lecture at college.

Jim and I had been long time friends at Eshton School. He was a budding geologist at heart and an amazing sportsman. He won the sprint races on Sports Day, was a gifted soccer player, and actor. He played the role of Dr. Faustus brilliantly in one of our annual school plays. He captained the school cricket team and left Eshton School in 1958 to attend Imperial College London to be trained as an expert geologist. He and his Canadian wife June traveled the world extensively, found many productive gold mines as well as other valuable metals in various continents, and finally settled in Tucson, Arizona, where they were blessed with a family of a boy and a girl, who have also traveled the world.

After one year at Mrs. Moxon's, I moved into Wilson House just off the Edgewear Road. Wilson House was named after one of St. Mary's Hospital Medical School Deans who was physician to Sir Winston Churchill and who was instrumental in making "Mary's" one of the top medical schools in the United Kingdom. St. Mary's Hospital was one of several medical schools in the capital city of London. As mentioned above, its claim to fame was its discovery of the antibiotic penicillin by Sir Alexander Fleming. Another Nobel Prize was awarded to Professor Porter of the Department of Pathology for his outstanding work on the immune system.

St. Mary's Hospital Medical School was also well known for its outstanding performance on the rugby field. Several players were selected to represent England in the international arena. An annual event was the London Inter-Hospitals Rugby Cup Competition, which St. Mary's either won or was runners-up. In 1973, the competition final was between St. Mary's and St. Thomas's Hospital. It was a great game, and I believe St. Thomas's won by a very narrow margin. The night before the game, we went to St. Thomas's Hospital School of Medicine, and I painted "Mary's for the Cup!!" with two exclamation marks afterwards on several locations. As the painting was being completed, a police car drove up and parked next to the footpath on my side of the road. Four members of the force got out of the car, two of whom were holding back a couple of massive Alsatian barking dogs. They left after I explained the situation to them, pulled their dogs into the police car, and drove away amused.

The next day, we drowned our sorrows at our local pub and after some nine pints a piece (there being nine supporters in our group), we somehow managed to get home in one piece, stopping on several occasions to decrease the volume of fluids on board!

During the time I was a medical student at St. Mary's Hospital School of Medicine, I made many friends. One group that immediately springs to mind was the Pandora Society and its select members. These included Nigel Evans (famous pediatrician) with whom I kept in close touch and was his best man at his unforgettable wedding party. His finance Patricia, a St. Mary's nurse, whom he met on the Pediatric Ward at a baby's cot, where it is believed she cried out, "Oh Doctor, I'm in trouble!" and Dr. Evans replying, in an Indian accent, "Well, goodness, gracious me!" as in the movie, *The Millionairess* starring Peter Sellers and Sophia Loren made some 60 years ago.

I regret to say that on Sunday, August 9th, 2021 at 11:00am Pacific Time, Pat, Nigel's wife, called that following a bout of acute cholecystitis, followed by endocarditis of an artificial aortic valve, Nigel passed away. This was a tremendous shock to all who knew him and our sincere condolences to his wonderful family.

Peter Latto, a fine squash and billiards player, who was nicknamed Q after the long wooden stick specifically made to play his favorite game of billiards.

Other friends included Alan Burr, John Whittingham, David Foster and Graham Moore (a fine cricket player), Jeff Glazer (who became a consultant surgeon at St. Mary's Hospital), Peter Beck, Bruce Henderson, Dick McPherson, George Morrison, and several others who became members of the Society later on in our student days.

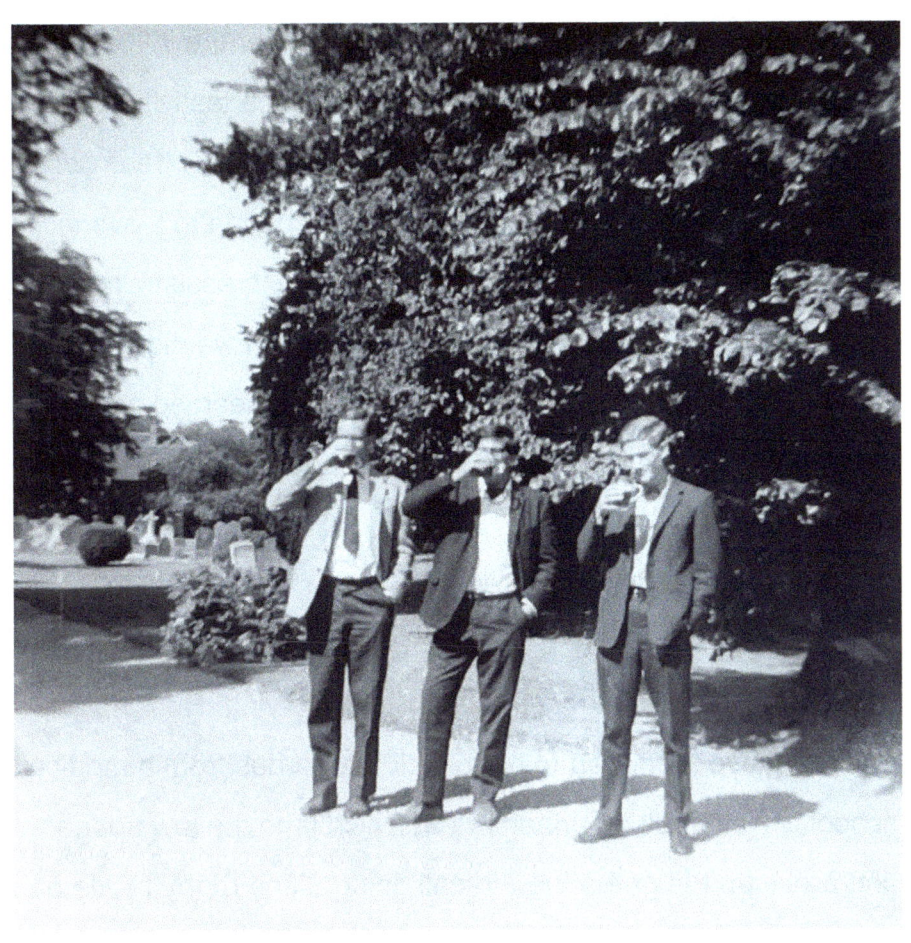

"Quenching Thirst." From right to left, Peter Latto, my brother Reza, and Nigel Boobyer.

St. Mary's hosted many clubs, one of which was the hockey club. Each club at St. Mary's had an annual festival. Dr. Jerry Grange was in charge of the hockey team. Accordingly, he made arrangements for a ball to be held to celebrate this occasion. A troublemaker made a point of attending all St. Mary's gatherings. On this occasion, he was well under the influence of alcohol when he showed up at the hockey team festivities and began to let off loud fireworks in the dance hall. This behavior was not appreciated by the supporters who began to leave in considerable numbers. Dr. Grange asked me to assist him in throwing out the culprit into Praed Street, which we did with pleasure. The troublemaker's colleagues who seemed as inebriated as himself came out in their friend's support.

A fight broke out in Praed Street, the police were called to restore order, but before their arrival, several supporters of our easily identifiable culprit came out with fists flying. Ducking and retaliating, we managed to beat back the hordes from a medical school, which shall be unnamed, at which time the law appeared and broke up the gathering. I recall doing a fine rugby tackle on the drunken fool who had started the whole disturbance and was flying down the Mary's main entrance steps going with intense determination at Jerry Grange's midriff. However, my tackle upset his rhythm as he went flying head first onto the cement floor!

The last member of the Pandora Society, but certainly not least, was Nigel Boobyer with whom I traveled through Europe and several countries behind the Iron Curtain after graduation. Nigel

Boobyer (consultant orthopedic surgeon) was nicknamed "The Colonel" because of his height, stature, and speech as if he was barking out orders!

After the final exams in 1964, we decided to take a trip together. He and I crossed the English Channel by car-ferry and traveled through France, Luxembourg, West Germany, and then south along the coast road in Yugoslavia which ran along the Adriatic Sea. The scenery was quite magnificent as was the city of Dubrovnik. We then traveled along the east coast of Greece taking in Thermopile (the site of the epic battle between a handful of Greeks and the vast army of the Persian King Xerxes), Marathon, where we climbed the hill made by Greek soldiers buried there following the Battle of Marathon between the armies of Greece and Persia. It is believed that the news of the Greek victory over the Persians at Marathon was carried by a Greek soldier who ran some 26.2 miles from the site of the battle to Athens in record time and collapsed at the end of his monumental feat!

We managed to drive to Athens that same day and were fortunate to find a nice apartment that evening. In Athens, we explored the Parthenon and several other monuments and took in the 'light and sound' show on the evening of our second day there. I recall that the Colonel and I stood up and cheered (much to the annoyance of the rest of the audience) when the announcer mentioned that it was Xerxes who had invaded and burnt Athens to the ground in 480 B.C.

During our stay in Athens, we had the pleasure of having Reza join us. He traveled from London to Athens by train and we met him at the Athens Main Railway Station. His journey was comfortable but boring. Reza is a person with a wonderful outlook on life and has a great sense of humor. He told us many jokes on our journey back to the UK and we were in good spirits all the way back to London.

On the last day of our stay in Athens, we decided to go for a swim. We drove to the beach, jumped into the Mediterranean Sea, and were delighted to see several young ladies arrive for a swim where we were. We plucked up the courage and started a conversation during which we discovered that the young ladies were employees of the British Embassy in Athens. We invited them to an imaginary party at our apartment that evening at 8 pm. We believed that they would not show up and therefore, made no effort to invite others and there was very little in the way of alcoholic drinks.

The girls arrived on time and there was an immediate chill in the air when they discovered that they had been tricked to an imaginary party, where instead of music, lots of people, plentiful drinks, there was absolutely nothing! They were upset at this deception and wanted to go home. Several of the girls lived in an apartment and they took their leave in their own car, and we had to transport the remaining girls to their homes. Needless to say, it turned out to be a disappointing evening, but it gave us an opportunity to pack our belongings for continuing onwards with our journey.

The next day, we headed for Crete. A crane was needed to lift the car onto the deck of a medium-sized boat. We slept on the deck next to the car to make sure no one tampered with it during the overnight sail.

We explored the island and were enchanted with its superb scenery. The beaches were of pure white sand against a backdrop of clear blue water of the Mediterranean Sea. It was a joy to be able to swim in it.

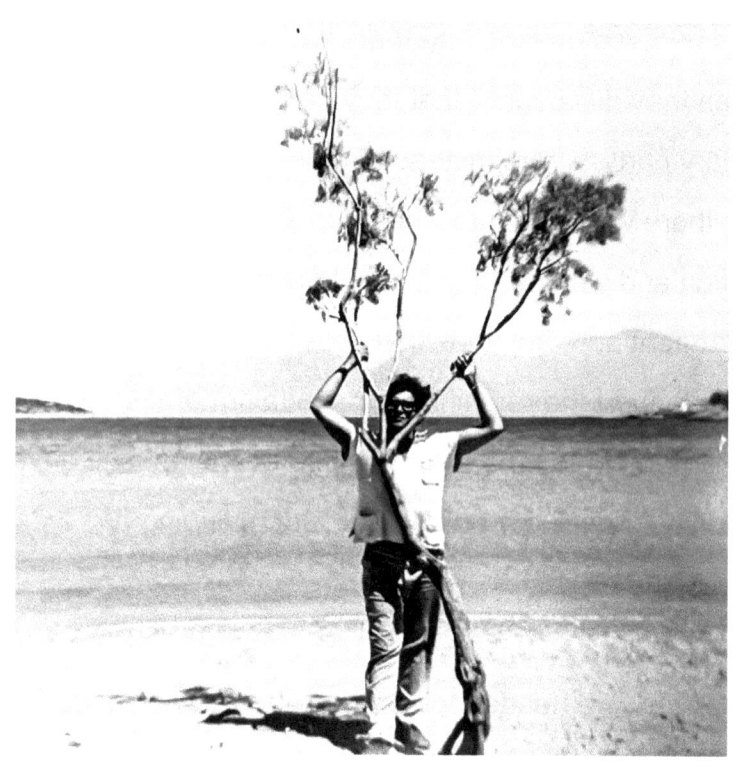

My brother Reza at the beach in Crete, Greece.

We returned to the UK via Bulgaria, Romania, Austria, and Czechoslovakia (where we gatecrashed a joyful party, walking through the open door of a house playing loud rock and roll music which enticed us to join unhindered from the street to chat up the girls). We got to northern France via East and West Germany, where we returned to the UK by a large car-ferry.

Unfortunately, Nigel lost his life in a tragic motor vehicle accident. He died instantly and his two daughters, who were wearing safety belts in the rear of the car, survived following a six-months stay in the ICU. I met his wife Mary-Louise many years later at a party in my brother's house, where, without my knowledge, a gathering had been arranged by Fereshteh, my sister-in-law, to celebrate my fiftieth birthday. Mary-Louise looked well and had remarried and was proud of her two daughters who had no post-accident problems.

After a "hard day's work," as per the Beatles' song, it was customary for members of the Pandora Society to gather at a pub in Lancaster Gate to imbibe several pints of beer and then cross the road to an Indian restaurant called "The Shahbaagh" (the King's Garden) for a curry. Being somewhat tipsy, we sang songs in a loud voice and on several occasions, the Colonel slipped his hand into the rice bowl and scattered the contents in all directions. The behavior of the group was such that after several complaints by the restaurant's regulars, the manager adamantly refused to let us be served the restaurant's hot, tasty curries anymore!

Chapter 3:

The Doctor - Patient Relationship

*"Much have I learned from my teachers,
more from my colleagues, and from my students
more than from them all."*

In 1964, after several months of intense study, the final exams came and went and all of a sudden, I was in demand for locum work (with pay!) having been granted by the University of London the MB BS (Bachelor of Medicine, Bachelor of Surgery– the equivalent of an American MD degree).

Then followed the house jobs (internships) in medicine for six months (at Paddington General Hospital) under the tutelage of Dr. Young and another six months learning surgery under Mr. Eastcott (surgeons were labeled as mister rather than doctor) and Sir Arthur Porritt, who was surgeon to the Royal Family. The Surgical Internship at St. Mary's Hospital was enjoyable, but the first six months as a medical house officer at Paddington General Hospital was tremendously stressful so much so that I seriously considered giving up medicine and hopefully going back to Eshton School to apply to become a member of the teaching staff.

An example of the stress level experienced at Paddington General Hospital (during my first internship rotation) was the frequency of waking up at night, thinking that the phone had rang and my presence was required in the emergency department where patients were lined up for admission. I would get up, wash, dress, and go down to the ER looking for the first patient to be evaluated for admission. The ER Staff would be surprised and amused, and after kind explanation that I had been dreaming, returned me to my quarters!

Each house officer was provided with a hateful pager that would buzz incessantly. One would have to use the telephone to determine who needed one's services. These included the causality department (ER), for admissions, senior staff of one's own team, colleagues, concerned ward staff, patient relatives, out-of-hospital calls, and most urgent of all, cardiopulmonary arrest at any site in the hospital.

Occasionally, one was presented with a problem that seemed Herculean and usually to a house officer's limited knowledge and experience, not solvable. Most of the patients under my care as a medical house officer had strokes, diabetes, or heart failure due to ischemic cardiomyopathy. Gastrointestinal bleeding usually due to peptic ulcer disease was a frequent cause of admission. The bleeding was usually due to the intake of NSAIDS or aspirin. COPD was seen fairly frequently because of excessive smoking. I also looked after a young Indian man with endocarditis of a bicuspid aortic valve. He was given a variety of antibiotics which were not effective in curing his disease (nowadays, he would have been cured by replacing his diseased aortic valve with an artificial one or a pig valve).

One of the cases that I remember vividly was a young man who was admitted with an extensive anterior myocardial infarction[1]. He was in bad shape (pale, sweaty, hypotensive, and anuric) when I saw him. He was being examined by me, and I had gotten to the neurological exam, checking lower limbs muscle strength by asking him to bend and straighten his left knee as hard as he could. He did what I had requested, and there being no intensive care unit (ICU) in those days with constant monitoring of MI patients, became unconscious and stopped breathing because of cardiopulmonary arrest.

---

[1] *Myocardial Infarction:* A heart attack.

In those days (1964), there was no or minimal training in BLS (Basic Life Support) and no training in ACLS (Advanced Cardiac Life Support). I was panic-stricken and asked the senior nurse what I should do. She paged the on-call anesthesiologist, my senior registrar, and the surgical doctor on call. Of course it took a substantial period of time for the team to assemble on the ward. The patient was intubated and someone attempted external cardiac massage. There was no response on the part of the patient. At this time, the senior surgical registrar decided to do a left-sided thoracotomy[2] and performed direct cardiac massage, all to no avail.

The presence of an ICU with cardiac monitoring and a readily available defibrillator might have saved this man's life. Doing an extensive physical exam, including performing a complete and rigorous neurological exam, doesn't seem, in retrospect, to be such a good idea.

In the early 1950s, I got my first view of a television set, the screen showing members of the Royal Family on the Buckingham Palace balcony. I remember watching the coronation of Queen Elizabeth II on television in 1953. Until then, we had the radio and listened to broadcasts, but this was the first time we saw something on the television that was of

---

[2] *Thoracotomy*: A cut in between the ribs to open up the chest. The doctor puts his hand inside the chest cavity and applies direct cardiac massage to the heart.

importance. Later on, whilst at Eshton School, the students gathered round the only television set in the establishment to watch Roger Bannister run the mile in under four minutes, the first person in the world to achieve such a feat! Every day, they replayed this scene, Bannister running the mile under four minutes, and we all gathered during our lunch break to rewatch this tremendous feat. He was at Cambridge University at that time and went to St. Mary's to study medicine and stayed on as a consultant in the Department of Neurology. He was knighted by the Queen for his achievements.

Sooner rather than later, every household in the land was blessed with a TV set, and now we are in the age of computers. Soon, computers had taken over the world, including the patient's paper chart. Rapid availability of patient data overtook the tedious task of finding the patient's paper chart! However, I recall the day that an elderly patient complained bitterly about the doctor no longer being interested in looking at the patient; rather, he was focused on the computer screen showing the various lab data. The days of the doctor-patient relationship had almost gone.

Super-specialization had taken over, so that making an appointment to see my orthopedic physician for a painful knee joint due to degenerative joint disease as well as address the pain in my left hip required two separate appointments to be made--one to see the orthopedic specialist for my knee, and another to see a different orthopedic specialist for the pain in the left hip region. Multiple X-rays of the painful area would have to be taken, followed by a visit to the new hip specialist.

Prior to this tremendous shift in medical practice, one could visit a single physician for these issues. However, I was told over the phone that I could not see doctor so and so for my hip if I had trouble with my knee, requiring two separate appointments, two separate bills, and two separate doctors, unified only by the data on the electronic medical record. How medicine had changed!

The following vignette illustrates this point:

Vignette for The Society of General Internal Medicine (SGIM)
California Regional Meeting
UC - Irvine
March 13, 2003

Submitted by:
Dr. Abbas Sedaghat
Professor of Medicine and Chief, General Internal Medicine & Geriatrics
VA San Diego Healthcare System

Title: The Indispensable Role of the General Internist in the Evaluation and Management of Complex and Puzzling Cases

Sub-specialists know a great deal about a limited number of topics. General Internists on the other hand are expected to know a substantial amount about all aspects of the vast field of medicine. The former are usually looked up to whereas the latter are often passed off as 'just general practitioners'.

The case submitted for presentation is one that illustrates the clear cut superiority of General Internal Medicine over the sub-specialties when it comes to complex and puzzling cases. Such cases occur with surprising regularity, are passed off by 'specialists' as 'not in my field of expertise' and discarded to be sorted out by the internist.

An elderly man walked into the VA Medical Center for cataract surgery. After the operation he was unable to move his limbs, stand or walk because of pain. The orthopedic team was consulted and after multiple x-rays, which showed no fractures, was diagnosed with 'arthritis pain'. The pain consultant was asked to see the patient. 'Myofacial pain and arthritis' was said to be the cause of the patient's symptoms and analgesics were recommended. The patient was transferred to the medicine service to receive PT (Physical Therapy) and Tender Loving Care (TLC). Evaluation of the patient by the internal medicine team revealed no muscle weakness, no muscle tenderness, a normal neurological exam and severe pain in all limb muscles on attempted movement. He had no headache and no new visual symptoms. A diagnosis of Polymyalgia Rheumatica (PMR) was made, confirmed by a sedimentation rate of over 100 and a dramatic response to small doses of prednisone over a few days. A temporal artery biopsy was negative.

This is an instructive case for those in the field of general internal medicine and illustrates the absolute need for well-trained generalists in this age of super-specialization.

Overdoses were commonplace mainly with barbiturates[3] and occasionally with aspirin. Once in a while, the pink appearance of an unconscious patient indicated carbon monoxide poisoning. Oxygen administration was the standard treatment as we had no access to a hyperbaric oxygen chamber[4].

The six-month surgical internship was essentially making sure that the patient was well enough to withstand the surgical procedure. My main function as a surgical intern was running back and forth to the Hematology Department to bring to the operating theater bottles of blood and ordering postoperative analgesia[5]. I also had to assist the surgical consultant who was an expert vascular surgeon and frequently operated on stenotic atherosclerotic lesions[6] in the femoral[7] and carotid[8] arteries.

---

[3] *Barbiturates*: Medical terminology for sleeping pills.

[4] *Hyperbaric Oxygen Chamber:* A procedure where one lays in a chamber, and instead of breathing air that is 70% nitrogen and 21% oxygen (which is what we normally breathe in), one breathes in 100% pressurized oxygen.

[5] *Postoperative Analgesia:* When patients come round from the anesthetic, one provides the patient with morphine for pain.

[6] *Stenotic Atherosclerotic Lesions:* Arteries narrowed by cholesterol deposits that build up in the arterial wall.

[7] *Femoral Artery:* An artery in the groin and in the thigh.

[8] *Carotid Artery:* The main artery in the neck that takes blood to the brain.

At the end of my six-month surgical rotation, I was extremely pleased to be complimented by the surgical team's senior registrar as the best intern he had ever worked with!

Not being sure of the specialty I wanted to follow and having made friends with several anesthesiologists during my surgical rotation, I was selected to become a senior house officer in the department of anesthesia. It was a fun rotation and I learned many anesthetic techniques from preparing children for tonsillectomy to preparing patients for attempted replacement of leaking abdominal aneurysms. The latter procedure was difficult, but our surgical unit accepted all cases in the London area. Most were unsuccessful, and I remember the renal resident in the OR wings during these operations wanting to see whether the kidneys were salvageable for transplantation into renal failure patients!

As an anesthetist, I was frequently on the cardiac arrest team. On one occasion, the call involved the arrest of a patient on whom I had performed an appendectomy[9] as a farewell reward at the end of my surgery internship. Supervised by my attending surgeon, the procedure went well, but post-operatively, he developed fever, for which no obvious cause could be found.

---

[9] *Appendectomy*: Removal of the appendix.

The cardiac arrest I had been called for was this young patient of mine who did not survive resuscitation. Autopsy revealed generalized venous thrombosis[10] with a massive pulmonary embolism[11]. It was a sad situation worsened by the difficulty of having to inform the very dejected family about the passing away of their young son. He was in his early twenties. I was asked by my Chief to stay on in anesthesia as a career, but I had the itch to participate in other medical specialties.

An application to the obstetric and gynecological department at St. Mary's Hospital failed. The consultant of that service who served the Royal Family, Mr. George Pinker, told me to apply elsewhere rather than stay at my alma mater to see what went on in other places within the vast field of medicine. He said that as fortune would have it, a Professor Walker, Chief of OBGYN at Queens University in Dundee, Scotland, was physically present at St. Mary's, acting as an external examiner, and was looking for a senior house officer to work in his unit. I met the professor that same day, the meeting was straightforward and after a couple of minutes, the professor asked me, "When can you start?" A month later, I was greeted on the grounds of Dundee

---

[10] *Venous Thrombosis:* Blood clotting in the veins.

[11] *Pulmonary Embolism:* When a blood clot in the legs moves up into the pulmonary artery, stopping the flow of blood to the rest of the circulation.

Royal Infirmary by one of the registrars (Chief Resident) who showed me the OBGYN unit and my lodgings.

For the first six months, I was SHO (Senior House Officer) in the gynecological department where there was no undue excitement taking care of patients with threatened abortion, performing D and C surgery in the operating room in cases of excessive bleeding in incomplete abortion cases. During my early days, I got to know a fellow SHO who befriended me and went on to become a consultant in OBGYN. I heard later that he had become President of the Royal College of Obstetricians and Gynecologists in London at the end of which period he was made Lord Patel.

Naren, as I called him, was a good friend to me. We often worked together. He was senior to me and often helped me out when the going got tough. We played cricket on the grassy area outside the doctor's dining room. We joked with Betty, who served us at meal times. She was a hard worker and a good friend to "her doctors," as she called the house staff.

Naren (Dr. Patel) had a relaxed attitude towards life, had a girlfriend who resided many miles away. He and I drank a small amount of single malt at The Bothy, followed by a few pints of bitter, before retiring to our rooms, a short walk from the pub. On one occasion, we decided to travel to East Germany to visit a Professor famous for taking a small blood sample from a blood vessel on the scalp of a baby who had difficulty in being delivered.

He measured the blood PO_2[12], PCO_2[13], Ph, and the lactate levels[14]. The data indicated whether an immediate C-section was required to save the baby (low PO_2, high PCO_2, and high lactate levels) or there was ample time for natural delivery to proceed. Having witnessed the procedure, we thanked the Professor and his team, and proceeded to Dortmund (a city in northern Germany) and nearby areas to taste the world-renowned beers of the region!

During that rotation, I got to know Dr. Booth Danesh, who was doing his PhD on an experimental lung and kidney machine. He and I became life-long friends, met frequently, and traveled

---

[12] *PO_2:* Partial pressure of oxygen, measuring the amount of oxygen in the blood. If PO_2 goes down, it means there is less oxygen going to the baby.

[13] *PCO_2:* Partial pressure of carbon dioxide. For a normal baby being delivered, it should be in the normal range. But if there are problems, the PCO_2 goes up.

[14] *Lactate levels:* A substance produced in the body when there is difficulty with the lungs exchanging carbon dioxide for oxygen. The oxygen goes down, CO_2 goes up, and it means something is wrong. PCO_2 in water is carbonic acid, and it is accompanied by the production of lactic acid. It has a normal range--if the baby is in trouble and needs a C-section to get it out of the uterus, the lactate level climbs to abnormal levels.

extensively together on the European continent. One of the memorable sights we visited in southern Spain was the beautiful Alhambra, a relic of the Islamic conquest of Spain many years ago.

On this journey, we traveled in Dr. Danesh's car (a comfortable Saab) and took in Sevill's impressive mosque and spent several days in Madrid. We then proceeded west to Portugal's capital city of Lisbon, at which point we flew to Majorca, a splendid island to the east of Spain in the Mediterranean Sea. There was a large contingent of tourists on the island. However, we had the advantage of being hosted by the parents of a friend of mine who worked in the emergency room (ER) at St. Mary's Hospital. She insisted that we should visit them in Majorca and gave us a detailed map on how to get to their residence. We were treated royally, put up for the night, taken to a fine restaurant where we had a wonderful serving of paella! The next day we tried our skills at water skiing, at which we failed miserably! The whole experience was memorable except for a single setback--I left my passport in Majorca on returning to Barcelona, Spain! This was resolved by our hosts in Majorca who sent the passport to the Iberian office in Barcelona on the very next flight. This was very kind of them, and their generosity to Dr. Danesh and I will not be forgotten. We were back in the UK in a couple of days via Catalonia, France, and the English Channel.

Dr. Booth Danesh was a replica of Omar Sharif, the star of Dr. Zhivago and Lawrence of Arabia. He was handsome, charming, and knew how to handle females who were attracted to him as bees to a beehive. He married a charming lady, Avril (also a doctor), and they have three wonderful boys, the eldest of whom became a famous entertainer.

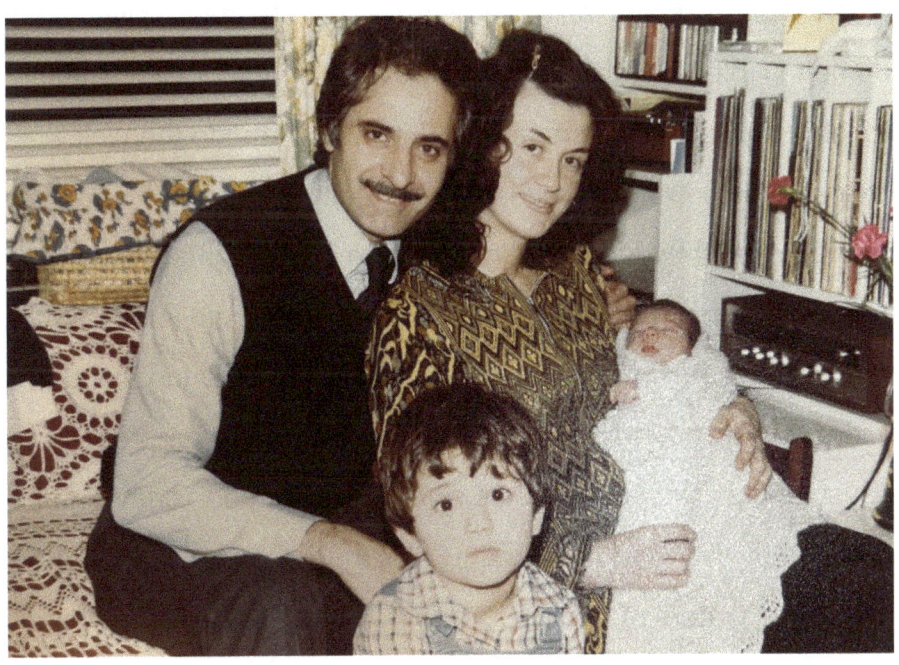

Dr. Booth Danesh, his wife Dr. Avril Danesh, and two of their three boys in Dundee, Scotland. January 1974.

My adventures with Dr. Danesh continued whilst I was visiting my sister, Gohar, in Tehran. I got a call from Dr. Danesh saying that he was planning a trip to Dubai for a week, and he invited me to join him for several days. Not having been to the Emirates before, I decided to join him, and accepted his invitation. I flew by Iran Air to Dubai. The Dubai Airport was modern, spotless, and well-organized. There was no need for a visa (for I had an Iranian passport which was acceptable to the authorities), and I was whisked through immigration without any delay.

A rental car was available, and I drove it to the impressive Jumeira Hotel, where I waited for several hours for Dr. Danesh to join me. Several beers at the "British Pub" made the wait tolerable! Following breakfast the next day, Dr. Danesh and I drove to the crowded city center to take in the sights. The city boasts a large Iranian population. Lunch was chelo kabab at one of the many Iranian restaurants, followed by a trip along a wide waterway winding through a fine city of many impressive skyscrapers. The next day, we swam in a fine pool, one of many boasted by the hotel, followed by a plunge into the clear blue and warm waters of the Persian Gulf, just a few meters away from the hotel pool.

A short walk away from our hotel was the magnificent sail-shaped Burj Al Arab--the only seven star hotel in the world! Whilst waiting for Dr. Danesh, I walked into this hotel, which was beautifully made and staffed by beautiful ladies carrying bowls of rose water on which floated magnificent roses for the guests to dip their fingers in. On the 17th floor was a helicopter pad, which was used by the Sheik and his guests to walk into their luxurious private suite without being pestered by the general public.

On my return to the Dundee Royal Infirmary and the six months of gynecology, I switched to the busy Obstetric Unit. Two events remain in my memory. The first was a ruptured gravid uterus, where the patient was in severe pain (put down to labor pains), where abdominal palpation revealed easily palpable fetal head, limbs, and body. My registrar and I had been on call and at work all the previous day and all that particular night. The consultant did rounds the next morning and carried out an emergency C-section to deliver a healthy baby boy, which had worked its way through a rupture (tear) in the uterus. Two things were evident: first that too long in the way of hours on duty was detrimental to obvious and correct diagnosis and that uterine rupture with the baby floating about in the peritoneal cavity was a condition to consider when baby anatomy was easily palpable on abdominal examination.

One night when I was on call for the Obstetric Unit and fast asleep, the telephone rang, and the labour ward sister told me that a patient had just been admitted with a prolapsed umbilical cord[15]. She was at term, but a prolapsed cord and its contents, the umbilical artery and vein, are very sensitive to temperature change, both vessels going into spasm and cutting off the blood supply to the placenta. This results in fetal hypoxia. Unless delivery of the baby is immediate, the fetus will die. Immediate cesarean section was needed to save the baby from hypoxia[16]. The nursing staff had placed the patient on a gurney with her body in the Trendelenburg position (head down, legs elevated) to prevent the fetal head from pressing the umbilical cord against the pelvic outlet. A moist warm towel had the prolapsed cord covered and there I was not knowing what to do next.

---

[15] *Prolapsed Umbilical Cord:* When a pregnant woman is in labor, the baby comes out first, and circulation in the umbilical cord continues to keep the baby oxygenated. Sometimes, however, the umbilical cord comes out first and as the baby follows it, its head and shoulders press the umbilical cord against the pelvis and cuts off the circulation; moreover, if the umbilical cord comes out first, its high sensitivity to temperature change can cause it to go into it spasm, resulting in a decrease in the circulation between the baby's blood and the mother's blood in the placenta, which can cause the baby to die, unless you can get it out quickly by C-section.

[16] *Hypoxia:* Lack of oxygen.

At that moment of ignorance, the registrar arrived on the scene to save the day (night). We got blood cross matched and put up an IV and prepared the operating room for an immediate cesarean section. To our horror, the consultant anesthetist lived some distance away and would be over half an hour getting to the hospital. The registrar who was all dressed and ready to go ahead with this necessary operation seemed impatient and distressed. I approached him and asked if I could anesthetize the patient for the surgical procedure. He recalled that I had just completed a year of anesthetic training at St. Mary's Hospital in London and nodded in agreement.

I pushed into the IV the appropriate dose of barbiturate[17] which put the patient to sleep followed by succinylcholine[18] to paralyze the patient so that I could intubate her. This procedure accomplished, I gave her curare to relax her abdominal musculature and nodded to the surgeon to proceed. He did so and delivered a healthy, crying baby. I reversed the action of the curare, so that the patient could breathe on her own, removed

---

[17] *Barbiturate:* A drug that is used for patients who have epilepsy that suppresses the activity of the brain and prevents the severe muscular activity in patients; a short-acting barbiturate can also be given into the vein to immediately put the patient to sleep.

[18] *Succinylcholine*: A drug that paralyzes the patient; the whole muscular system becomes paralyzed. It is given to the patient, so that one can easily put the endotracheal into the trachea.

the endotracheal tube, and gave her some morphine to dull the pain of her cesarean section.

It was at this moment that the operating room door flung open and in walked the elderly anesthesiologist on call, furious that someone else had beaten him to the anesthetic procedure. He calmed down when he had been informed that I had been trained by several anesthetic consultants at St. Mary's Hospital who were friends of his. Everyone seemed happy and satisfied, and word soon spread in the hospital that Sedaghat, the OBGYN SHO, had saved the baby by anesthetizing the patient. I became quite famous!

It was customary for all members of the Department to gather in the local pub called the "Bothy" at the end of the working day. On one occasion, I asked one of the departmental consultants (Dr. Jack Crawford) how to get involved in a rugby club to get some exercise. Within a couple of weeks, I was contacted to play for a team at the fly-half position[19]. My opponent was an agile and speedy young man, who scored a try within minutes of the start of the game! It was my job to stop him from scoring. So whenever the opposition had the ball from a line-out or a scrum,

---

[19] *Fly-Half Position:* During a rugby match, when the scrum-half puts the ball between the two teams who are bent over and pushing against each other, if the scrum-half then receives the ball, he usually passes the ball off to the fly-half, who then can run with it or kick it ahead, or passes the ball to the inside center, outside center, and finally the wing.

I started my run to knock my opponent down by hitting him with my shoulders just above his ankles every time he was given the ball!

On one occasion, towards the end of the game, I knocked him down with my head instead of my shoulder, following which I do not recall anything other than being led off the field, directed to the changing room, and being driven to the Dundee Royal Infirmary by a variety of considerate team members. I presume this was a case of concussion!

The next adventure I ventured into was a one-year rotation in the Department of Pathology at St. George's Hospital at Hyde Park Corner in London's West End within walking distance of the world-famous shopping center Harrods. The rotation involved clinical chemistry for three months and three months learning histopathology (looking at microscopic sections of organs and biopsy specimens). It was not a very enjoyable rotation and I am not too sure I got any major benefit from it. The site of the hospital, now a luxury hotel, was its saving grace, being across the road from Hyde Park Corner and several historical monuments of interest, including the residence (now a museum) of the Duke of Wellington (victor in a major battle at Waterloo against Napoleon Bonaparte of France in 1815).

For a period of six months, I was sent to a part of St. George's Hospital in Tooting, London, about one half-hour drive from Hyde Park Corner. It was a regular general hospital and I spent half of my time in the hematology department and three months in the bacteriology section of the Institution. Dr. Fleck, who ran the bacteriology department, was a world authority on toxoplasmosis[20]. This organism is transmitted to humans via the cat and can cause fetal damage in the pregnant patient.

One night when on call at the hospital, the medical resident brought in a blood sample from a Nigerian patient who had been admitted in a comatose state. The history revealed that he was on his way back to the United Kingdom following a business trip to the Middle East. The plane had made a ten-minutes landing at Abuja in Nigeria to drop off some cargo, at which time the plane doors were open. A sample of the patient's blood was prepared and stained in the usual manner and on high field microscopy showed red cells packed with Signet's Ring Trophozoites[21]. On scanning the field, gametocytes were noted

---

[20] *Toxoplasmosis:* A parasite carried by cats. When cats defecate, the toxoplasma comes out with the feces, and if it contaminates the food or drink, the person who has had contact with these organisms becomes infected.

[21] *Signet's Ring Trophozoites:* When the red blood cells that carry oxygen to the tissues and remove carbon dioxide via the lung become infected with the malaria parasite, the cell becomes big because it's loaded with trophozoites, and occludes (blocks) the blood vessels, particularly those that flow to the brain. With no blood flow to the brain, the patient goes into coma.

as well, making the diagnosis of the patient's coma one of infection by plasmodium falciparum malaria[22], probably following a mosquito bite during the plane stop in Abuja. This illustrates the importance of a careful history, including the travel history, in all sick patients.

During my year at St. George's Hospital, I prepared myself to take part in one of the MRCP (Member of the Royal College of Physicians) examinations of the United Kingdom. I passed the written portion of the exam during my stay at St. George's Hospital, but had difficulty in the face-to-face patient evaluation on two occasions.

---

[22] *Plasmodium Falciparum Malaria:* There are four different types of malaria--Plasmodium Falciparum Malaria kills by obstructing blood flow to the brain.

Chapter 4

Specialization

~

"Climbing the Ladder"

To get promoted in the field of internal medicine, one had to pass the MRCP examination. The examination consisted of two parts: the first was the written component followed by an interaction with a chosen patient whose issues had to be taken care of. To be successful in getting the "membership," as it was called, it was necessary to obtain as much experience in clinical medicine as possible. This meant completing my SHO post at St. George's Hospital and finding a position at a busy hospital as a Registrar (Chief Resident). Several attempts proved unsuccessful until my discovery that a Registrar's position had become available at my own teaching hospital—St. Mary's! Without any hope of success, I decided to give it a try and applied for the post.

At the time of the interview, I found myself in a waiting room filled with several familiar faces, including the Gold Medal Winner in Medicine at St. Mary's Hospital, several years my senior. The familiar faces were in my year or above, all with impeccable backgrounds and achievements superior to mine!

I felt foolish to try and compete with such outstanding candidates and was about to leave the scene when Dr. Cockburn, the medical superintendent at St. Mary's Hospital, invited me to the interview room. Several personalities were recognized instantly, including Dr. Young, Mr. Eastcott, Sir Arthur Porritt, Dr. Cockburn, and one or two who I had never encountered previously. The interview went fairly well, and to my utter amazement and pleasure, Dr. Cockburn grabbed my arm on our way out saying the unbelievable words, "You have got the job!" Surprise, disbelief, pleasure, elation, happiness descended upon me, and I remained motionless for some considerable time to absorb what had just happened. I then rounded in the hospital with pride and joy, telling anyone who would listen of my unbelievable achievement!

It was at this time that I was informed of MRCP courses held by Dr. Maurice Pappworth preparing candidates for the second part of the membership examination. I joined his course, read his excellent book, *"A Primer of Medicine,"* on how to approach the patient encounter with confidence and picked up advice that I had never been given before and which I use to this day to teach my medical students and residents with success. His approach was to take a complete history and whilst doing that, observing the patient and his surroundings for things, such as the administration of oxygen and the presence of an IV infusion, how the patient struck one on first being seen, noting his skin color, the pattern of his breathing, the severity of his pain, followed by a complete physical examination, including inspection, palpation, percussion, and auscultation[23]. He pointed out that having a complete history and carrying out a full physical examination, the candidate should have a list of the differential diagnosis. He also taught us how to interact with the examiner, not to allow prolonged pauses during the discussion of the case, and to enumerate the differential diagnosis for the examiner without hesitation.

As mentioned above, I was able to pass the MRCP exam after three attempts, clinching a diagnosis of hyperthyroidism[24] in a male patient on my third attempt. This success was due to hard work and assistance in the technique of discussing a difficult

---

[23] *Auscultation:* The stethoscope is used to listen to the lungs and the heart sounds, searching for any abnormalities.

[24] *Hyperthyroidism:* Overactivity of the thyroid gland in the neck.

case with the help of Dr. Pappworth. The latter was an outstanding teacher of clinical medicine who taught me as well as thousands of other candidates how to present a patient to the examiners in the MRCP exam. His style was impressive and one that I copied in my later career as a teacher of clinical medicine to university students and residents at the University of California, San Diego, where I was Head of the Division of General Internal Medicine and Geriatrics at the Veterans Affairs Medical Center.

As a Registrar at St. Mary's Hospital in London, my attendings were Dr. C. Young, a diabetic expert with vast knowledge and experience in this important field as well as medicine in general and Dr. W. Brooks, CBE FRCP, who was a generalist with a special interest in diseases of the chest. As a Registrar to the above consultants, I had a Senior Registrar and two excellent House Officers with whom I worked. Every fourth day, I was on call for medical care of patients coming to the Emergency Room and who were admitted as necessary.

Several observations whilst an in-patient because of glandular fever[25] promoted my knowledge of internal medicine. I was

---

[25] *Glandular Fever:* A disease where the patient has a sore throat, fever, with cold-like symptoms as well as enlargement of lymph nodes in the body. It is due to infection by the Epstein Barr virus.

hospitalized for several weeks, where some evenings, I noted difficulty breathing, which improved when Dr. Cockburn gave me a course of ampicillin, which for unclear reasons improved my sore throat and made my breathing easier.

While laying in the hospital bed, I observed a case of sickle cell disease in a Jamaican man who was admitted in considerable pain due to priapism[26] induced by his Sickle Cell disease. Other cases seen by me with this disease included a woman who presented with hemoptysis (coughing up blood). Chest X-Ray revealed an area of consolidation. It was the hematologist who diagnosed the Sickle Cell Disease by looking at a blood smear[27] in this patient. I also saw a young boy later on in my career when I was in Shiraz, Iran, who presented with severe tibial bone pain in his left leg, which was thought to be due to Sickle Cell Disease[28], resulting in bone infarction.

---

[26] *Priapism:* When the penis enlarges because of the sickle cells obstruct the return of blood from the penis back into the general circulation. The enlargement becomes extremely painful.

[27] *Sickle Cell Disease Blood Smear:* When you look at a blood smear in people with Sickle Cell Disease, the red blood cells look like a sickle (an instrument used by farmers to cut down plants that grow high).

[28] *Sickle Cell Disease:* Sickle cells occlude the blood vessels preventing red blood cells from carrying oxygen to the tissues, and if it involves the bone vessels, it results in great pain due to bone infarction.

Shortly after returning to work, I was presented with a patient who was a boxer and who had been knocked out the night before in a boxing match. He had recovered consciousness, but prior to admission to the hospital, he went into coma again. No neurological findings had been noted when he came round following his knock out and had returned home.

The next morning, he was found to be in coma. X-rays of the skull showed no fractures. A spinal tap was carried out looking for hemorrhage in the sub arachnoid space[29] from a brain injury (on reflection, this was the worse procedure to carry out in these circumstances!)[30]. He was transferred to the neurological unit at Great Ormond Street. He died shortly afterwards. The autopsy revealed an intracerebral hemorrhage resulting in increased intracranial pressure with resulting coning of his brain stem into the foramen magnum[31]. A few days later, a patient in coma was admitted and was found to be in renal failure[32]. He was admitted

---

[29] *Sub arachnoid space:* The space between the brain tissue as well as the spinal cord and the bony canal that surrounds the brain and the spinal cord.

[30] *Spinal Tap*: This involves pushing a needle in the back in between two vertebral spines, usually between the third and fourth lumbar vertebrae, with the purpose of removing fluid from the spinal column to give you information regarding what's going on.

[31] *Foramen Magnum:* This is an opening in the skull, where the brain joins the spinal cord.

[32] Renal Failure: A condition when the kidneys have stopped working.

for peritoneal dialysis[33]. He recovered from his coma and was transferred to the renal transplantation unit next door.

I got a call from the ER Head Nurse one day to evaluate a Jamaican lady in her thirties who had arrived with severe lower abdominal pain of sudden onset several hours prior to coming to the hospital. My visit was short and to the point. She was late in her periods for several weeks, was not on the birth control pill, and had taken no precautions against becoming pregnant. Examination revealed a lady in severe pain. She had pale mucous membranes, had tachycardia[34], and a low blood pressure. Abdominal examination revealed little movement of the abdominal wall with tenderness and guarding in the left lower quadrant. I was unable to hear any bowel sounds. Pelvic examination was painful for the patient. The pain became worse on moving the cervix. Bi-manual examination revealed a mass the size of a tennis ball on the left side of the pelvis. The

---

[33] *Peritoneal Dialysis (PD):* A condition carried out in people with renal failure. The kidney's function is to get rid of all the unwanted materials in the body. In renal failure, there is no excretory function, keeping all the unwanted things in the body. The PD treatment involves making a hole in the abdominal wall to allow a catheter through which 1-2 liters of fluid (usually sodium chloride and other solutions) are put into the peritoneal cavity, following which the caterer is clamped and left for a couple of hours. What then happens is that unwanted materials, usually exerted by the kidneys, are excreted in the fluid in the peritoneal space. After two hours, one reverses the flow, applying pressure to the abdomen, thereby removing the fluid with the unwanted materials.

[34] *Tachycardia:* Rapid heart rate.

pregnancy test was positive and thus a diagnosis of an ectopic pregnancy[35] with rupture of the left fallopian tube was made.

An emergency call went out to the intern and senior registrar of the OB-GYN department stating that the patient was in need of excision of the left fallopian tube as well as removal of the left ovary. A blood sample had already been sent to the laboratory for grouping and cross match of several units of compatible blood, and the transfusion was started. The fame of a medical registrar with exceptional diagnostic capabilities at St. Mary's Hospital had begun!

Several other cases of interest encountered in the emergency department included a middle-aged gentleman with acute onset of abdominal pain with board-like rigidity on abdominal examination, absent bowel sounds, and air under the diaphragm on abdominal X-ray examination (erect view). His perforated duodenal ulcer healed well after emergency surgery and suturing of the perforated site.

A further case of interest was the admission of an elderly patient with seizure-like activity. He was unconscious with no response

---

[35] *Ectopic pregnancy:* In normal pregnancies, the fetus is in the womb. Sometimes, the actual baby that is developing gets bigger and bigger in a place outside the uterus, and this is often in the tube called the *fallopian tube*, which connects the uterus to the ovary.

to external stimuli, no focal neurological signs were detectable, his pulse was very slow, and his blood pressure was unrecordable. The electrocardiogram revealed marked bradycardia (slow pulse at a rate of some 15 beats per minute) and evidence of complete heart block. The exam was otherwise normal and there was no response to several doses of IV atropine (a medicine, when given to a patient, speeds up the heart rate). The cardiac registrar was called and preparations were carried out for putting in an intravenous wire catheter to pace the patient. He was paced at a rate of 65 beats per minute and within a few moments, he was awake and telling us jokes as he was transported to the cardiac unit. He did well with a permanent pacemaker put in the next day.

My two years as a Registrar at St. Mary's Hospital came to an end in 1970. Those years were the most enjoyable time of my career mainly because of being with my brother Reza, meeting and becoming friends with his Queen's University Belfast associates, and falling in love with Theresa who was one of the medical students at St. Mary's Hospital School of Medicine. I took advantage of my access to London's concerts, theaters, and the opera (introduced to me by my dear friend Dr. Nigel Evans).

I shared an apartment with my brother in Holland Park in London, where we threw parties regularly, at which time champagne (the Real McCoy) was served whilst munching on French bread and cheese, and enjoyed each other's company. My brother Reza, four years my junior, was at Eshton School with me. He went to college at Queen's University in Belfast Northern Ireland and graduated with a degree in Geology.

Several years later, he obtained a Master's degree in Geology. Later in his career, Reza went on to obtain his PhD in the field of Geology from Imperial College of the University of London. Initially, he was interested in going to work in Canada for any one of several oil companies. However, my father insisted that he return to Iran, work in the southern Iranian oil fields with the Oil Consortium Organization, and be of service to the country of his birth.

It is appropriate here to mention that all Iranian men in the 18-30 years of age group were expected to do military service for four years. Reza was drafted into the military on his return to Iran in 1969. His command of Farsi (the Persian language) was minimal and he found military service extremely difficult.

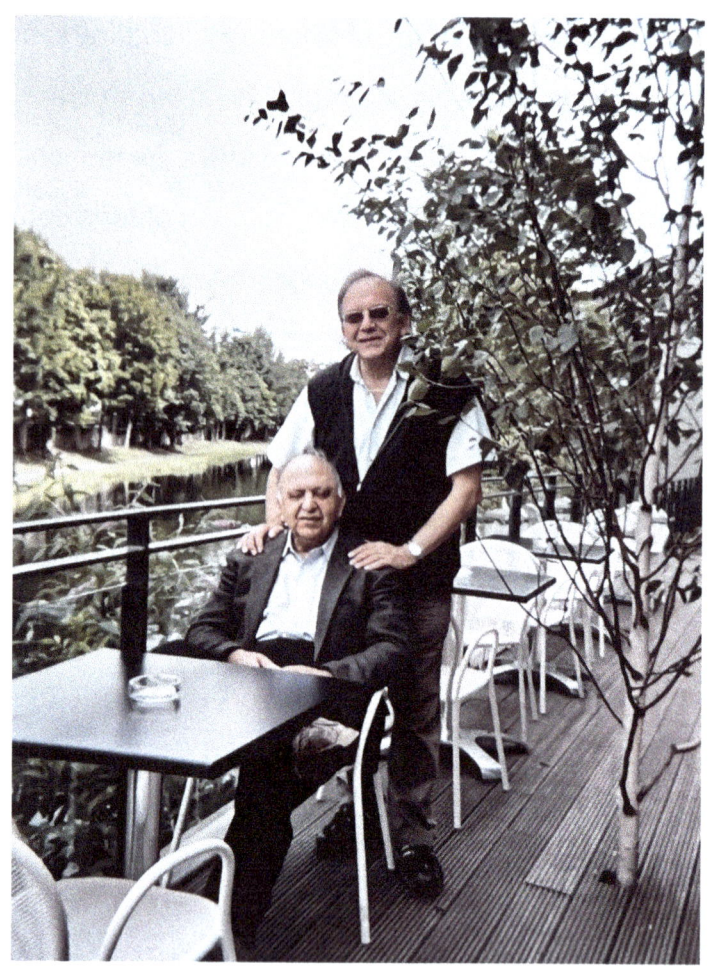

My brother Reza and I relaxing by the river Thames in London, England.

His commanding officer took advantage of Reza's British credentials and he was asked to tutor senior officers in the English language, which he did for several years. After four years, including two years in the tank corps in Shiraz as part of his military service, Reza married an Iranian lady by the name of

Fereshteh. Following the birth of a cute son (Ali) and a beautiful daughter (Maryam), the family decided to move to the UK.

The Khajar Dynasty was a corrupt and incompetent one, and during this period of time, large oil rich areas of the country north of Azerbaijan were absorbed into the Soviet Union. Meantime, Iran was divided into areas of influence by a variety of tribes including the Ghashghais, the Kurds, and the Lor tribes in the west, and the Turkeman and Baluch and Bakhtiars in eastern Iran.

Ingrid and I visited the Ghashghais camp in the summer of 1977. We were served tea in the traditional Iranian hospitality way. The tribe moved south towards the Persian Gulf during the winter and migrated north in the summer to the cooler region of the country passing by Shiraz and Mashad in the northwest towards the picturesque Alborz Mountains. We purchased a fine colorful carpet made by this tribe woven on a horizontal loom. In the 1930s, there emerged an Iranian soldier, a member of the Cossack Brigade in the north of the country, who was a patriot and wanted a unified, disciplined, and self-sufficient country free from foreign influence. He took charge of his regiment and began to stop tribal rivalries, corruption, and detrimental activities by force when necessary. He was crowned Reza Shah

Pahlavi and stopped activities which had kept the country a backward nation for so long. He kept Iran a neutral nation during the Second World War. The Allies, for questionable political reasons, stepped in, banished him from his beloved country and deported him to a variety of destinations in the African continent until his death in Egypt. He was replaced by his son Mohammad Reza Shah Pahlavi. Reza Shah's body was returned to Iran in the late 1940s. I remember going to my father's pharmacy in Pahlavi Square and standing on a chair behind the front of the pharmacy, which was all glass, to see the historic event. Thousands of Iranians turned out to pay homage to this great man, who played a major role in modernizing Iran. His body was placed in a mausoleum in the holy city of Ghom, which we visited on several occasions. Following the religious revolution in 1979, the mausoleum was desecrated because anything to do with Royalty was destroyed. At that time, the religious government expelled the Shah and his family from Iran and began to rule the country with an iron fist.

Once my brother Reza left, I missed him a great deal, but work and studies filled the void. During my rotation as a Registrar at St. Mary's Hospital, I managed to obtain the MRCP (Member of the Royal College of Physicians), a necessary and difficult degree to obtain.

Chapter 5

BTA: Been to America

"We don't have Scurvy in America!"

At that stage in my life, I was ready to return to my country to be of service to it as my father had wished. Having lived in the UK for 21 years, my knowledge of Farsi (the Iranian language) was meager, and I was not familiar with the customs and beliefs of most of the Iranian population. At that time, following a discussion with my father regarding my future, he pointed out that most medical personnel who were successful in Iran had had some sort of training in the United States. I decided to discuss this issue with Professor Peart.

Professor Peart was an outstanding clinician and researcher in charge of the whole Department of Medicine at St. Mary's Hospital Medical School. It so happened that he was a good friend of Dr. Alex Bearn, Chairman of the Department of Medicine at New York Hospital Cornell Medical Center in New

York City. As luck would have it, several telephone calls within a period of two days secured me a teaching residency position at New York Hospital Cornell Medical Center, and within a couple of weeks, I was on a plane bound for New York City!

The journey was uneventful, and on arrival at the hospital situated on the upper eastside of this vast and vibrant city of New York, I was met by Frances "Tim" Weld, the Department of Medicine's Chief Medical Resident, a knowledgeable, kind, and understanding physician, who showed me to my quarters and the relevant parts of the 25-floor hospital (there was a tennis court at the top of the hospital building, which was in great demand by the house staff). The next two years at Cornell was an eye-opener for me. I was the resident on the 15th and 16th floors, where well-to-do and famous persons from the nearby United Nations (UN), such as the Shah of Iran, TV celebrities such as Johnny Carson, etc. were taken care of.

A bunch of dedicated medical students followed me on our daily rounds, where I became known as a desirable teacher of clinical medicine.

A case of miliary tuberculosis[36] with meningitis[37] stands out in my mind as a case I diagnosed and got credit for. I was very impressed by the pains taken by the Institution to provide a substantial amount of time for lectures, conferences, tutorials, etc. for the house officers. I participated fully in these sessions and often offered to cover for others in various departments during holidays and special occasions. A novelty was playing or trying to participate in baseball with the house staff and playing rugby with a team of medical students!

I had five senior medical students in my team, all bright and keen to learn as much medicine as possible. They were kind and generous and often invited me to their homes for dinner. One of the five was a female who objected strongly to the male dominance in the medical field. Having got to the door leading to the library, I opened it and kept it open until all the students had gone in. The last person to enter the library was the female medical student who said that she was able to open the door herself and keep it open for all to pass through, and she was in

---

[36] *Miliary Tuberculosis (TB):* TB is transferred from person to person by droplet infection via the lungs similar to COVID transmission. The droplets get into the lungs and set up foci of infection. Sometimes, the infection involves the whole body, and little foci of tuberculosis spread throughout the lungs and elsewhere throughout the body.

[37] *Meningitis:* Inflammation of the tissue covering the brain and the spinal cord.

no need for acts of chivalry by the male sex to have the door opened and allow the ladies to go through first!

I took the opportunity to explore New York City, took walks in Central Park, and began enjoying New York City's massive pizzas and hamburgers. Full advantage was taken of operatic performances at the Metropolitan Opera House, and concerts at the nearby New York Concert Hall at the Lincoln Center. The Russian tea house became a favorite of mine for refreshments. New York is a fabulous city, and I enjoyed my four years there immensely.

I recall volunteering to cover the emergency room over the Christmas season in 1971. The ER was not particularly busy as ambulances transported acute emergencies to other medical centers. One night, the ER staff asked me to evaluate an elderly man complaining of left thigh pain. During my conversation with him, it turned out that he was poor, and lived on tea and biscuits (cookies). Examination revealed a large hematoma[38] in the musculature of the left anterior thigh. There was no history of falls or other forms of trauma, so that the painful swelling in his left leg was spontaneous. Closer observation revealed

---

[38]*Hematoma:* A collection of blood.

perifollicular hemorrhages[39] and thus, a diagnosis of Scurvy was made. The admitting house officer was aghast at my diagnosis, stating, "We don't have Scurvy in America!" The patient was admitted to the hospital and was found to have a zero level of Vitamin C in his blood! He recovered fully following the administration of Vitamin C.

My ultimate aim was to return to Iran and join the School of Medicine in the beautiful city of Shiraz (situated in south-central Iran). The Shiraz Medical Center was set up and run by the University of Pennsylvania School of Medicine per encouragement of the Shah of Iran. Two major hospitals formed the core of the Pahlavi University Medical Center. One was built and funded by a wealthy Iranian businessman and patriot Mr. Nemazee. All medical students, nurses, and faculty (initially from the University of Pennsylvania) spoke English fluently and were replaced over the years by American-trained, Iranian personnel. Communication was in English. All charts and orders were in English and Pahlavi University Medical Center (PUMC) became well-known as the top medical school in the country.

---

[39] *Perifollicular Hemorrhages*: Throughout the body, there are little spaces called hair follicles through which the hair comes out. In Scurvy, which is due to Vitamin C deficiency, there is bleeding in the perifollicular regions.

To obtain a position at this medical center as a faculty member, one had to have carried out research and published a minimum of three papers in internationally recognized medical journals. I discussed my plans with Dr. Alex Bearne, who suggested that I stay at New York Hospital as a faculty member in Internal Medicine. However, I was determined to return to my country and asked for his opinion regarding getting involved in research work. A telephone call to Dr. Peter Ahrens, who was a leading figure in lipid metabolism, secured me a position in his laboratory at the famed Rockefeller University. The Rockefeller University, a renowned research center, with several Nobel Laureates amongst its staff, was situated next to the New York Hospital.

The following two years, I participated in lipid research with the help and encouragement of Dr. Ahrens. Several drugs were in extensive use at the time, including Atromid S and Cholestyramine. Using radio-active C14 (Carbon 14) and gas liquid chromatography, we were able to measure the level of Atromid S. We showed that the concomitant administration of these drugs did not interfere with the absorption of Atromid S, a medication used to reduce the serum cholesterol. We managed to publish several papers in well-known lipid journals including the *Journal of Clinical Investigation, Journal of Lipid Research,* and the *European Journal of Clinical Investigation.*

In the early 1970s, Dr. Grundy asked me to participate in a gallstone meeting in Chicago. Most of the speakers were Japanese and the presentations were about pigmented gallstones. Most gallstones are of the pigmented variety in Japan, in contrast to mainly cholesterol stones in the Western Hemisphere.

Chapter 6

The Return of the Prodigal Son

~

"Shiraz: The City of Roses and Nightingales"

The offer of a position as an associate professor at the Pahlavi University School of Medicine (PUSOM) came, and I embarked on my journey to Iran, visiting Rome, and Istanbul in Turkey, accompanied by my finance Ingrid (German-born American lady), whom I had met at the Rockefeller University. The large extended family group was at Tehran's Mehrabad Airport to greet me after an absence of 21 years in the UK and four years in New York City. Following a short stay at my parents' residence in northern Tehran, and a bewildering Iranian style marriage, I headed for Shiraz—the city of roses and nightingales—and the burial sites of two of Iran's world-renowned poets—Hafez and Saadi.

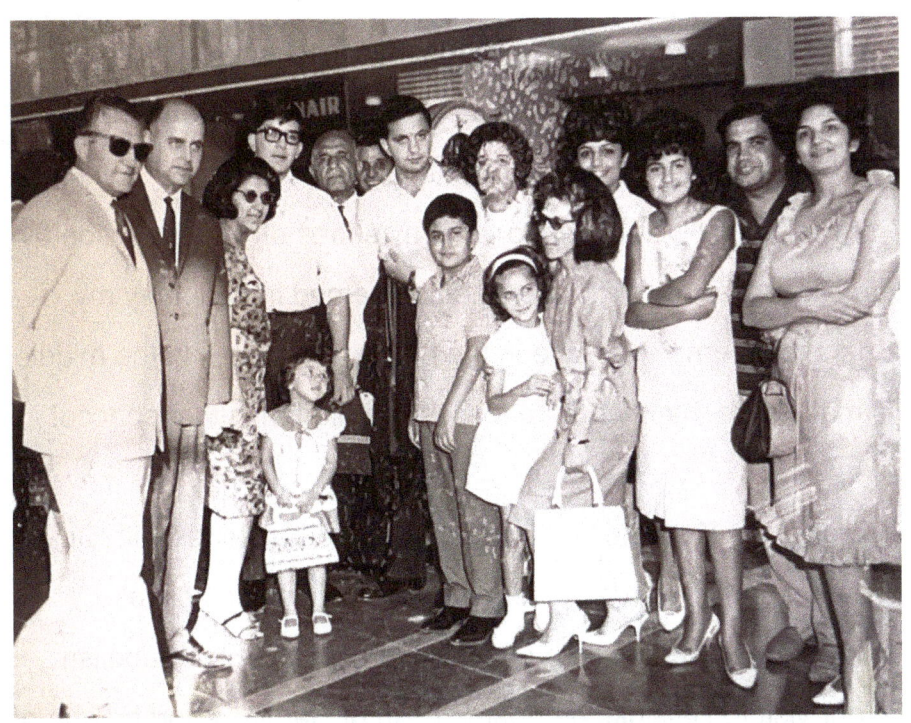

The extended family gathering at the Tehran International Airport to greet Reza, myself, and Sadegh (in the middle of the picture) after many years of training overseas.

During the four years (1974-1978) spent at the PUMC, we made a trip to Tel Aviv in Israel and one to Helsinki in Finland to present papers in the field of lipid metabolism. The trip to Israel was of interest. The conference was like any other I had attended before. The highlight of the visit was renting a car and taking in several Biblical sites, including the Wailing Wall, sacred to the Jewish faith, the beautiful Al-Aqsa mosque above it, where those of the Muslim faith prayed and where it is believed that the Prophet Muhammad began his journey to heaven on departing from this world. We visited Jerusalem, the birthplace of Christ, the founder of the Christian faith. On the way back from Tel Aviv, I was asked to take my shoes off for inspection by the airport security official who also seemed intrigued by my cigars, each and everyone in the box being broken in the middle to make sure there were no explosives hidden in the tobacco!

Whilst at the Rockefeller University, I became friends with Dr. Kesaneimi, a charming researcher from Finland who was studying the role played by the skin in cholesterol metabolism. In our visit to Helsinki, he hosted us in his family resort by one of the lakes draining into the North Sea. We spent some half an hour in the sauna followed by jumping into the lake. Heated by the time spent in the sauna, the cold water of the lake felt wonderfully refreshing. We rented a car and explored some of the splendid areas around Helsinki. My research paper presentation on the effects of the antibiotic neomycin on cholesterol metabolism was delivered well to several members of the audience; it being the last presentation on the last day of the conference. We attempted to visit the sights of St. Petersburg across the border in the Soviet Union, but were unable to get across for political reasons.

I made a name for myself as a teacher of clinical medicine to my house officers and medical students. The emphasis was on kindness and understanding towards the many sick patients and the importance of a complete and thorough history and physical examination followed by an in-depth discussion of the differential diagnosis. I observed tragic cases of rabies and tetanus, severe cases of myasthenia gravis[40] and multiple other conditions. One case of note was a young man with severe hypertension and associated hypertensive retinopathy, whose blood pressure hit rock bottom when he was given a dose of regitine[41]. His blood pressure became unattainable and he had to be resuscitated by IV fluids and placed in the Trendelenburg position. He was operated on and his pheochromocytoma[42] was removed successfully by our surgical team.

---

[40] *Myasthenia Gravis:* A disease in which the patient's muscles are partially paralyzed. They have difficulty opening their eyes. In severe cases, they have difficulty chewing or swallowing and have difficulty moving their legs. It is a neuromuscular disorder.

[41] *Regitine:* A substance that blocks the effect of epinephrine and norepinephrine, which constrict the blood vessels and keep the blood pressure up. If there is too much of these two agents being produced, usually by a gland in the abdomen called a pheochromocytoma in the posterior wall of the abdomen near the kidneys, then the blood pressure increases.

[42] *Pheochromocytoma:* A rare cause of hypertension (hypertension).

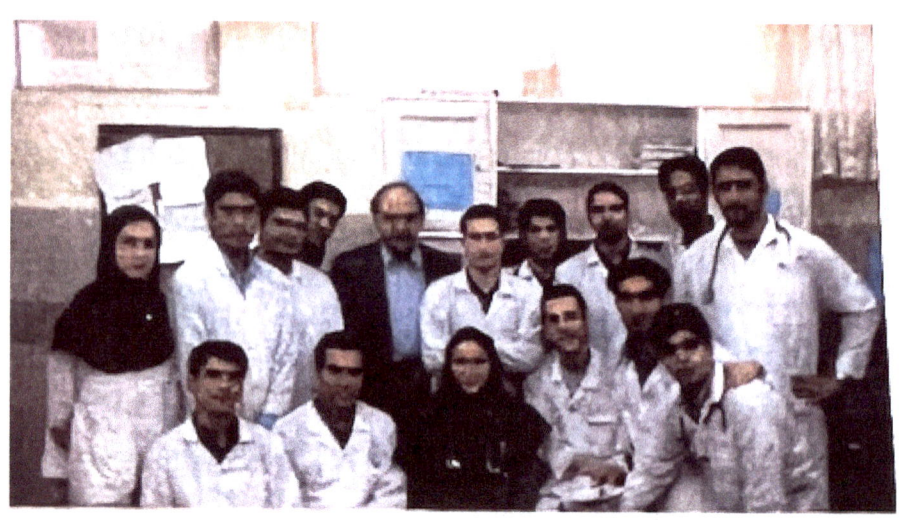

My residents and interns as well as students at Nemzee Hospital in Shiraz, Iran.

A case I failed to diagnose miserably was a young lady admitted to the Nemzee Hospital in coma, with a rapid pulse and unrecordable blood pressure. She was not on any medications, there was no evidence of bleeding, and she was not dehydrated. There were no clinical features of Addison's Disease[43] and other than the above findings, the physical examination was normal. She was not using tampons (thinking

---

[43] *Addison's Disease:* A condition where there is damage to the adrenal glands, which secrete hormones, including hydrocortisone and aldosterone.

about toxic shock syndrome[44]) and I could detect no skin rash (thinking about meningococcemia[45]). I wondered about hydatid cyst rupture[46] resulting in an acute allergic reaction. One thing I did not carry out was an EKG to see whether this was an arrhythmia causing her hypotension. This was done several hours later and showed ventricular tachycardia[47]. She recovered following cardioversion and was handed over to the Cardiology Department for further evaluation and treatment.

Most of the patients were poor and often brought to the Medical Center late in the disease process. Aplastic anemia[48] was seen frequently as were opioid overdoses in young and distressed members of the community. Several patients were lost, but a

---

[44] *Toxic Shock Syndrome:* A condition tied to contaminated tampons by staphylococcus bacteria that causes rapid pulse, low blood pressure, a feeling of light-headedness, which may cause loss of consciousness.

[45] *Meningococcemia*: An infection caused by the bacterium meningococcus, which causes a skin rash, hypotension, and often proceeding to death usually in persons in their late teens.

[46] *Hydatid Cyst Rupture:* Following infection with the hydatid parasite produced by worms which infect the body and become established in many organs, some of which form cysts. If the cysts rupture, an allergic reaction to the contents of the hydatid cyst may occur.

[47] *Ventricular Tachycardia:* A rapid beating of the heart, the contractions originating in the ventricles.

[48] *Aplastic anemia:* When the marrow doesn't produce what it's supposed to produce– which is red cells, platelets (a decrease in platelets may cause the patient to bleed), and white blood cells (to help fight off infections).

substantial number were saved by gastric lavage[49] and the administration of several doses of naloxone.[50]

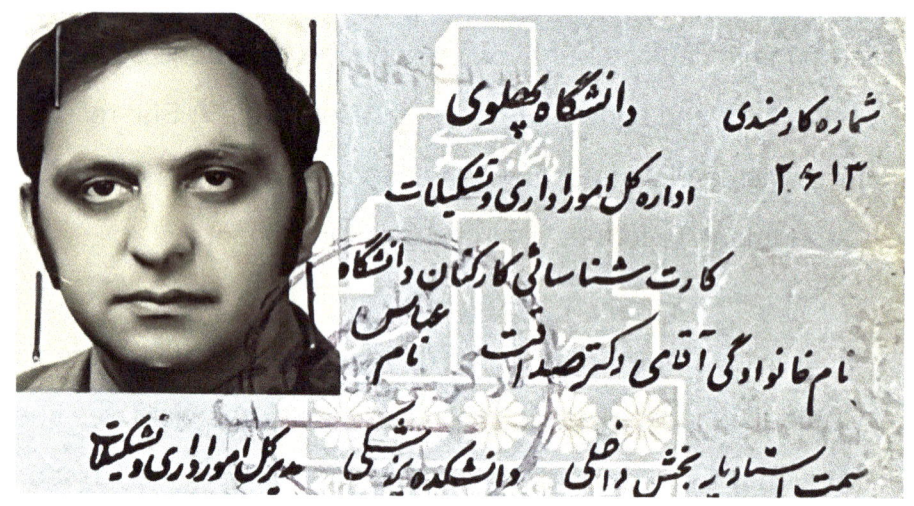

My Pahlavi University Medical Center ID Card in 1974.

Another case of interest was the lady with cholera who required 22 units of intravenous IV saline with added bicarbonate and potassium. This disease is endemic in Bangladesh, India, and is due to consumption of contaminated food and water. The organism responsible for the disease is a gram negative

---

[49] *Gastric Lavage:* When a tube is pushed down the esophagus into the stomach, and a funnel is put in one end of the tube, water or saline is poured in, filling up the stomach, mixing with the stomach contents. The funnel is then brought down to ground level, resulting in the stomach contents being removed by gravity.

[50] *Naloxone*: A medication that is an anti-optiate, so that if someone has taken, say, opium, by mouth, one can counteract the effects of opium on the body by giving them naloxone, an antagonist to morphine.

bacterium (vibrio cholerae) which stimulates the cells lining the GI tract to secrete water, sodium, potassium, and bicarbonate. Nausea and vomiting is uncommon in this disease, so oral therapy plays a major role in the treatment of epidemics of the disease. The WHO recommends the administration of water to which sodium bicarbonate, potassium chloride, and sodium chloride has been added.

An intramuscular (I.M.) injection of a vaccine for travelers to endemic areas is available, but only partially effective. Another common disease seen in the outpatient clinic was the bite of a sandfly, which can jump a distance of 12-15 inches. It is a bloodsucking insect that carries a parasitic organism called amastigotes and results in a papule followed by its enlargement and ulceration of the skin usually in the lower extremity. These lesions are disfiguring and usually heal following treatment with parenteral pentamidine[51] injections, leaving a disfiguring scar.

A visiting dermatologist from St. John's Hospital near Piccadilly Circus in London spent a year with us in Shiraz. He was an adventurous character and had heard of a mullah (a religious person) in Yazd who had concocted a cream that was supposedly highly effective in the treatment and cure of many

---

[51] *Parenteral Pentamidine:* A drug effective against a variety of diseases by worms or organisms injected into the body by mosquitoes.

with this disease. He, the dermatologist, and I using the Saadi Hospital car went on an interesting journey to find this mullah to provide us access to his magic cream to use at our dermatology clinic in Shiraz. The journey was an interesting one highlighted by the car being stuck in a riverbed, which we were trying to cross. In a short time, we were surrounded by a mass of people who pushed the car across the water with ease allowing us to proceed on our journey. One of our Pahlavi Medical Center (PMC) senior residents, a bright and kind gentleman, was in Yazd at the time and helped us to locate the mullah with access to the formula to his famous cream, which supposedly cured cutaneous leishmaniasis. The mullah was a wiley old man who had made a substantial income dispensing his "magic cream" to patients with this condition. He was not fooled by our offer of purchasing his chemotherapeutic agent, and we returned to the hospital empty-handed without even having the opportunity to see it or witness the effects of this concoction.

To take advantage of being in Yazd and unsuccessful in obtaining the magic cream to treat leishmaniasis,[52] we went to visit a nearby mountain of human skeletons at the Zoroastrian burial site on the outskirts of the city. Zoroastrianism is a form of

---

[52] *Leishmaniasis:* When a sandfly bites a person on the leg, and injects its organism, leishmaniasis is the disease that follows this injection. It starts off as a bump, followed by ulceration of the skin, which heals with scar formation.

religion now banned in Iran. When the people died, they were piled on to this hill-like affair, and pecked away by birds, so that all that remained were the bones.

Whilst in Shiraz, we made several trips to Tehran to visit the family. We would drive to Isfahan, spend a night in the beautiful Shah Abbas Hotel, dining on hamburgers in the gardens of the hotel before retiring. The next morning, we would have breakfast in the magnificent dining room adorned with chandeliers of exquisite quality before setting off for Tehran via Ghom.

We would arrive in the afternoon, warmly greeted by my father and his second wife Khanom Naficy, of the illustrious Naficy family whom we called "mom." The weekend trip was frequently spent catching up on the news of family and friends and trips to the "Villa" by the Caspian Sea. Many orange trees bearing an abundance of oranges adorned the garden. The Villa was situated in 'Shahsavar' next to the beach and not far from the charming town of Ramsar. Reza Shah the Great was instrumental in the creation of this jewel of a place. Running through the hotel and available to the guests were gigantic baths (big enough to swim in!), which could be filled with hot natural spring water with a pungent smell to soothe inflamed joints.

Another visitor to our Medical Center in Shiraz on a one-year sabbatical was Dr. Brian Creamer. He was a wonderful person, kind, considerate, and an outstanding physician with a special interest in diseases of the gut. On his return to London, he was made Dean of St. Thomas's Hospital School of Medicine and helped several of our attendings and senior residents who fled Shiraz at the time of the Iranian Revolution, when the Shah was deposed and the Islamic religious group came into power.

Other visitors to our Medical Center in Shiraz included Dr. Maurice Pappworth, Dr. Nigel Evans, and a good friend of ours from the Department of OB-GYN from Dundee, Scotland by the name of Dr. Jeff James. We also had a superb neurologist who spent several months teaching our students and house officers a substantial amount of neurology. She was a Professor of Medicine and Neurology at Columbia University Medical Center in New York City's upper west side.

Another trip of interest was a visit to an area northwest of Shiraz, where the food was deficient in iodine. There were multiple cases of goiters because of iodine deficiency. The addition of iodized salt to the diet of these patients was magically effective in normalizing the size of their enlarged thyroid glands. The enthusiasm for this adventure was Dr.

Mohsen Shahmanesh. Mohsen was an expert in diseases of the thyroid gland and had been trained at St. Thomas's Hospital in London situated just across the river Thames from the magnificent Houses of Parliament. Dr. Shahmanesh was treated poorly by the religious zealots in Shiraz at the time of the Revolution and was imprisoned in the infamous Evin Prison next door to the luxurious Hilton Hotel in north central Tehran. He fled to London with his wife and was helped by Dr. Brian Creamer to become a consultant in the clinic dealing with cases of AIDs and other sexually transmitted diseases.

Because of my experience in emergency medicine, I took charge of the ER at the Saadi Hospital and made efforts to streamline the process of evaluation, treatment, and immediate admission of emergency cases to various specialized units. Because each ER patient was accompanied by a substantial number of family, the ER was used as a holding ward, because of lack of in-patient beds and was frequently overcrowded by a massive number of patients, family, and well-wishers!

One of my achievements was the improvement of the ER functioning rapidly and smoothly. Unfortunately, this was not permanent and visits to the unit several years later when I visited Shiraz University Medical Center to participate in the teaching program, the changes I had laboriously made were not altogether well maintained.

A major attraction for visitors to Shiraz was the nearby archaeological site of Persepolis (the winter palace of the Achaemenid Kings such as Xerxes and related royalty). Not far from Persepolis was the historic tomb of Darius, the most famous of the Achaemenids. These sites were visited by the Pahlavi Medical Center Visiting Faculty as a must, and frequently, I was the person transporting them to these fabulous sites via a town called Kazeroon.

During my stay in Shiraz, I completed the composition of an MD thesis submitted to the University of London. I was requested to be interviewed by consultants at the Hammersmith Hospital in the 70s. One of the interviewees, a consultant nephrologist, objected that the thesis was too short and that there was no mention of the renal effects of the drug clofibrate on the kidney.

I was required to rewrite and resubmit the thesis, which I did, with many references to his own work in the field of nephrology. The thesis was accordingly accepted, and a copy lies in the University of London library in the UK.

In 1978, I had provided enough time and energy to be given a one-year sabbatical. At this time, there seemed to be student unrest and demonstrations against the Shah and the rest of the Royal Family. The monarchy came to an end, the Royal Family left Iran as a religious figure (Khomeini) returned to the holy city of Ghom in Iran and set up a religious theocracy which continues to this day.

For my sabbatical, I had contacted Dr. Scott Grundy whom I had met in Dr. Ahren's laboratory at the Rockefeller University in New York. Dr. Grundy had by then moved on to the University of California in San Diego, setting up his laboratory at the VA Medical Center. He invited me to work in his laboratory looking into the mechanism of gallstone formation. Our research was published in the *New England Journal of Medicine* in June of 1980.

December 12, 1978

The Editor
The Manchester Guardian Weekly
164 Deansgate
Manchester
England

Dear Sir:

    At a time when it seems fashionable to expound at length about the personality and questionable behaviour of the Shah being responsible for the present unrest in Iran, it was a welcome change to read the article by Martin Woollacott entitled "Shah: scapegoat for Iran?" (November 26).

    All men, including illustrious leaders of democratic nations, have their weaknesses and the Shah is probably no exception to the rule. The regime in Iran has made many mistakes and admitted to doing so.

    Unfortunately, however, almost all recent reports on Iran have omitted to mention the tremendous advances made by that country over the past 37 years under the leadership of the Shah. These include the implementation of the revolutionary land reform bill, the immense expansion in the provision of educational facilities and health care and, of utmost importance, the emancipation of women. In a backward country torn apart by the events of the second world war, on the verge of famine, bankrupsy and lawlessness, these accomplishments were no mean feat.

    The regime has been repeatedly accused of corruption. Although not to be condoned, corruption has been and will continue to be a way of life within all classes of Iranian society. It cannot and should not be blamed solely on the Shah.

    Martin Woollacott's article looks with rare insight into the reasons for repression in Iran. I quote: "Iranian society, left to itself, was likely to have produced an array of conflicting political forces ....." and "..... the Monarchy prevented the victory of any of them or, more likely, <u>a chaotic conflict</u> between them .....".

    It is my belief that the majority of patriotic Iranians feel that the Shah, whatever his failings or past mistakes, is the only able and experienced political leader who has the genuine welfare of his country at heart. Without him Iran will be a poorer nation - if indeed it continues as a unified country. There are many who feel that if the Shah were to abdicate Iran would be engulfed in civil war and probably disintegrate as a nation.

                                           Sincerely yours,

                                           Dr. A. Sedaghat

EXHIBIT 1B

Copy of a letter to the Manchester Guardian regarding the Shah of Iran at the time of the Iranian Revolution.

Chapter 7

Luxury Medicine

~

"From Research to Clinical Work"

During my time at the VA Medical Center, I volunteered to do attending rounds and teach ICM (Introduction to Clinical Medicine) to students who were finding the going somewhat difficult. The Chief of the VA Medical Center, Dr. William Hollingsworth, noted my interest in patient care in Internal Medicine, which resulted in my being invited to join the VA Faculty several years later.

With the generalized decrease in funding for research, I began to look for work elsewhere. A friend of mine recommended me to an attending physician at Scripps Clinic in La Jolla, California, who was in the process of recruiting well-trained physicians to create a division called "Community Medicine." This was in response to a rapid increase in the population of San Diego County, which continues to this day. I began work at Scripps

Clinic in 1980. The clinic was luxurious and provided services to the well to-do. Many patients came to seek reassurance that all was well by having check-ups. These were wealthy persons from Saudi Arabia, the Emirates, Mexico, Iran, and many from La Jolla in California. Most had the worried well syndrome and who underwent a series of unnecessary tests, reassured, and billed enormous amounts for these services.

I struck up a good working relationship with my colleague Dr. Anthony Moore, who was head of our section for years. He was an avid surfer and made annual trips to Fiji with some of his friends to ride the waves of the Pacific Ocean. He was a good internist, worked hard, but was faced with a difficult home life. In the late 1980s, on reaching the beach after an exhilarating surfing session, he collapsed and all attempts at resuscitation failed. I suspect he had coronary artery disease and ended up with a terminal malignant arrhythmia[53].

Dr. Parviz Foroozan, a kind and considerate gastroentrologist, who headed the division of gastroenterology and was an outstanding physician befriended me and was supportive during the years of turmoil when Ingrid developed severe depression

---

[53] Arrhythmia: When the heart rhythm goes from normal to either too slow, too fast, or becomes irregular.

with several attempts at suicide. This was in spite of God's gift of a son, Martin, who was born on June 19, 1981.

Ingrid's pregnancy was a complicated affair as she had antibodies to Martin's blood group. She was followed by a supporting team of OB-GYN personnel and was induced at 34 weeks. The baby, obviously premature, anemic, and jaundiced because of antibody induced hemolysis of his red cells, was kept in the pediatric ICU for several weeks after undergoing several exchange transfusions at that time. He is now a strapping young man with a family of his own and a wonderful teacher of English at a school in Niigata, Japan. Ingrid's depression, several hospitalizations at Sharp Hospital, ECT (electro-convulsive therapy, where they put the patient to sleep via anesthesia and pass an electric shock through the brain), my lack of close family support and concern about my own mental health led me to seek my brother's input regarding my own future. A speedy divorce and a move to London in the UK to stay at my brother's residence took place in quick succession in 1987. Martin was enrolled in a private school and was encouraged to spend his school holidays in San Diego with his mother.

During the eight years spent working at Scripps Clinic, several cases of interest were encountered. These included my first patient on day one, an elderly lady with a chronic productive cough, inspiratory rales over both lung bases as well as obvious clubbing of the fingers. She was referred to the chest clinic, which confirmed my diagnosis of bronchiectasis[54] by bronchography[55].

On a Saturday morning, I was called to see a man who, whilst gardening at home in Rancho Bernardo, was stung by an insect (probably a horse fly) over his right shoulder. The area became ulcerated and he developed enlargement of several lymph nodes on the right side of his neck. A clinical diagnosis of Tularemia[56] was made, confirmed by culture of the organism in the laboratory; he was given intramuscular injections of

---

[54] *Bronchiectasis:* the lung alveoli, where carbon dioxide and oxygen are exchanged, are destroyed. This results in shortness of breath, the blood oxygen falls, and carbon dioxide level increases.

[55] *Bronchography:* In this test, a radio-opaque material is introduced into the trachea, the bronchi, and the alveoli. and enters the right and left main bronchus, and outlines the lung tissues. X-Rays show dilated spaces of the area, which are not effective areas for oxygen intake and carbon dioxide removal.

[56] *Tularemia:* This is a disease that is transmitted to humans by the bite of a horse fly. The organism is endemic in squirrels and other animals in wooded areas. The horse fly bites these animals to get blood for nutritional purposes, and the organism in the fly is highly infectious, and it may cause skin ulceration and lymphadenopathy as well as pneumonia in humans.

streptomycin[57], which cured his infection. Interestingly enough, the patient's son came to see me with similar symptoms several weeks later. The diagnosis was made and treatment for infection with Francisella Tularensis[58] undertaken. This organism, a gram negative bracillus, is endemic in several animals (rabbits, squirrels, etc.) and is transmitted by bites of horse flies and deer flies from the infected animals to man. It is dangerous to handle in the laboratory because of possible infection of the bacteriologist.

Another case that was seen in the urgent care center was a middle-aged lady who had been to several ERs complaining of prolonged weakness and dizziness. She had been reassured that there was nothing wrong with her. My examination revealed pigmentation of her skin, including the buccal mucosa and gums, and a low blood pressure with significant postural hypotension. Her labs revealed anemia, hyponatremia[59], and hyperkalemia[60]. I diagnosed the case as one of Addison's Disease confirmed by the presence of a low serum cortisol,

---

[57] *Streptomycin*: This is an antibiotic that kills bacteria in diseases such as Tularemia, Tuberculosis, and other conditions.

[58] *Francisella Tularensis:* The name of the bacterium that causes Tularemia.

[59] *Hyponatremia:* A low serum sodium.

[60] *Hyperkalemia:* High serum potassium.

unmeasurable aldosterone, and no response to ACTH stimulation.

The difficulty in such cases is the diagnosis. Once it is made, the treatment is quite straightforward and includes oral cortisone and florinef[61]. I informed the department of endocrinology of the diagnosis, which was poo-pooed, but confirmed by appropriate laboratory testing. The diagnosis was poo-pooed because it is an uncommon disease and often missed as in this case. Prior to discharge from the clinic, a champagne party was given to which I was not invited. I presume this was because the Chief of Endocrinology at the Clinic felt that I was incorrect in my diagnosis when I telephoned him about the case and seemingly was embarrassed about his behavior.

A patient with pneumonia was admitted to the hospital. He had been seen by me previously. On taking the history, he mentioned that his son had just come back from South America and had brought some parakeets with him. The possibility of

---

[61] *Florinef:* A medicine given to patients that works by absorbing sodium by the kidneys and excreting potassium, the reversal of what causes Addison's Disease.

psittacosis[62] arose and was confirmed by serological testing[63]. This case impressed upon me the importance of taking a careful travel history.

In the early 80s, my friend, James (Jim) Mayor, came to visit us when we were living in Solana Beach in a fine house with a superb view of the ocean and magnificent sunsets when sitting in the garden on a bench looking west. During our conversation, he mentioned that he had a lump on the back of his hand over one of his metacarpo-phalangeal joints for which he had had recent surgery to have it removed. This was done under local anesthesia, and Jim mentioned the fact that when the surgeon dropped the lump he had excised into a metal bowl, it made a sound which he likened to a sound produced by metal on metal. I was intrigued by this statement and wondered whether the lump was composed of iron. Excessive deposition of iron in the body is a feature of hemochromatosis. I wrote a note to his doctor in Tucson, Arizona, that he should have his serum iron measured as well as the percentage of saturation of his transferrin. He called me several weeks later and said that my diagnosis was correct, and he indeed had hemochromatosis. To

---

[62] *Psittacosis:* An organism that causes disease in birds. Psittacosis is Latin for birds. When they sneeze, the organism is inhaled by humans and may cause a pneumonia.

[63] *Serological testing:* a blood test.

this day, he continues to have one unit of blood removed every month as therapy for this condition.

Shortly afterwards, I saw an elderly gentleman who had arthritis of both knees, excessive pigmentation of his skin, as well as an enlarged liver with abnormal liver function tests. His serum iron was high and his iron binding capacity was almost fully saturated. A high serum ferritin[64] clinched the diagnosis of hemochromatosis[65] for which he was treated by the removal of a unit of blood every month. The diagnosis would have been missed if the excessive skin pigmentation and a palpably enlarged liver had been missed by not performing a careful physical examination.

The importance of a complete and thorough physical examination was once again impressed upon me at the time an Iranian patient of mine with asthma came to the Scripps Clinic for a routine visit. On listening to his chest, a loud ejection systolic murmur was audible, which I had not noted on his previous visits. This murmur was best heard at the cardiac apex

---

[64] *Ferritin:* A test for this particular condition called hemochromatosis.

[65] *Hemochromatosis:* Is a condition where most of the iron in the food is absorbed by the gut. Some 99% of the iron is absorbed instead of 24%, which is the normal amount.

and radiated to the left axilla[66]. The differential diagnosis included: aortic stenosis[67], tricuspid stenosis[68], atrial septal defect[69], ventricular septal defect, mitral regurgitation[70] as well as a flow murmur. His asthma seemed under control and in passing, he mentioned that he had had dental work a few weeks prior to his visit. His chest X-ray was normal, and his CBC and his chemistry panel were unremarkable. He had a mild leukocytosis[71] as well as an elevated sedimentation rate[72]. Several blood cultures were

---

[66] *Left axilla:* The left armpit.

[67] Aortic Stenosis: When there is a narrowing of the aortic value through which the blood is pumped out of the heart into the general circulation.

[68] *Tricuspid Stenosis:* There are four valves in the heart. Tricuspid stenosis is a narrowing of the tricuspid valve, where the blood flows from the right ventricle through this valve to the pulmonary artery.

[69] *Atrial Septal Defect:* In the heart, there are two atria and two ventricles separated by a muscular wall. If there is an opening in the atrial septum, or an opening in the ventricular septum, there is a loud murmur when listening to the heart, between the first and the second heart sounds.

[70] *Mitral Regurgitation:* Occurs when the mitral valve is defective. Normally, blood flows from the left atrium into the left ventricle. If it is incompetent, a systolic murmur is audible due to blood flowing from the left ventricle back into the left atrium.

[71] *Leukocytosis*: An increase in the white blood cells, due to infections, usually bacterial infections.

[72] *Sedimentation Rate:* When a blood sample is put in a fine tube and left for an hour, the red cells and the white cells come down the column (they're heavier than the serum), so in the hour, they measure how quickly that column increases as the red and white cells settle down. If they go down rapidly, that's a high sedimentation rate, which is the case in a variety of infections.

taken and a cardiac echo was arranged. The next day, my infectious disease colleague called me at home saying that all blood culture bottles had grown strep viridans[73]. The patient was asymptomatic and did not know what all the fuss was about. The cardiac echo revealed mitral valve prolapse (MVP) but no vegetations[74]. He was admitted to the hospital and started on IV penicillin, switching to oral agents after several days. He made an uneventful recovery after a week in the hospital and continued on oral antibiotics for several weeks after discharge.

The lessons learned from this case include: one, antibiotics are indicated in dental manipulations in those with MVP; two, mitral valve prolapse (MVP) may be present without any findings on physical examination; three, outpatient oral antibiotics should be considered after several days of inpatient IV antibiotic administration; four, consider SBE (subacute bacterial endocarditis[75]) in patients with new onset cardiac murmurs; five, SBE may be totally asymptomatic in some patients.

---

[73] *Viridans:* A bacterium that is in the mouth. If dental work is carried out, this bacterium gets into the blood circulation, and once in the circulation, the bacterium may end up on the mitral valve area, making the mitral valve insufficient, resulting in a systolic murmur.

[74] *Vegetations:* Clumps of bacteria growing on the valve cusps.

[75] *Subacute Bacterial Endocarditis*: A condition in which bacteria attached to valve cusps resulting in inflammation of the heart valves.

In contrast to the above was the tragic case of a lady in her early twenties who came to the urgent care center in shock (blood pressure unrecordable), a sore throat, fever, and a generalized erythematous macular rash[76]. She complained of headache and neck stiffness. Meningitis was confirmed by a spinal tap, IV antibiotics were administered as well as large doses of steroids and vasoconstrictors. She died in the ICU within 24 hours and autopsy and bacteriology findings were compatible with meningococcemia[77]. Vaccination early on would have prevented her death.

Weekly grand rounds were held at the clinic. Dr. Moore and I did a presentation entitled, "The Uncommon in Community Medicine." We discussed several cases we had seen in the clinic, and were awarded the Best Grand Rounds for the year of 1983-1984.

---

[76] *Erythematous Macular Rash:* Erythematous means red, and a macular rash is something seen on the skin which is not palpable, so the patient sees a series of red spots on the skin.

[77] *Meningococcemia:* A bacterium that is often fatal in young people, around college age, within 24 hours.

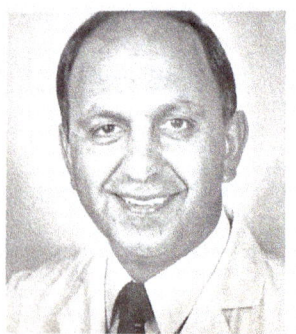

Dr. Abbas Sedaghat

Abbas Sedaghat, M.D., Division of Community Medicine, has been elected a fellow of the Royal College of Physicians of the United Kingdom in recognition of his services to medicine including teaching and research accomplishments. Sedaghat obtained his medical degree from the University of London where he also received postgraduate training in anesthesiology, obstetrics and gynecology, pathology and internal medicine. He subsequently received further training in internal medicine at Cornell University Medical Center and did research work in lipid metabolism at the Rockefeller University in New York. Prior to joining Scripps Clinic in 1979, he was visiting associate professor of internal medicine at University of California San Diego Medical Center where he continued his research work in lipids.

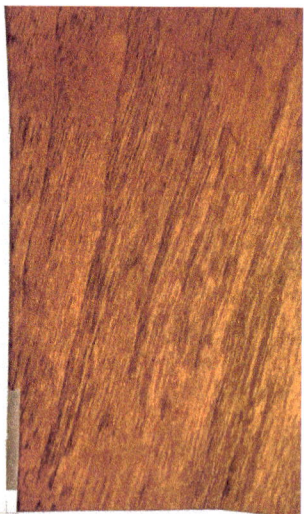

A note in Scripps Clinic's monthly newsletter regarding my involvement with the Division of Community Medicine in 1985.

Other diagnoses of interest during my time at Scripps Clinic included a case of toxic shock syndrome associated with the use of staph aureus (a common bacterium) contaminated tampons, a middle aged man with glandular fever who returned to the clinic with an acute abdomen several days after the initial diagnosis and who was found to have a ruptured spleen, an uncommon complication of Epstein Barr virus infection. Other cases diagnosed at the clinic included a young man with a history of hemorrhoidectomy[78] who returned for evaluation of an extensive Erythematous Skin Rash including the palms of his hands. A diagnosis of secondary syphilis was made and confirmed by reexamination of his hemorrhoidectomy slides using a silver stain[79], which showed the classic spirochetes[80] of syphilis[81]. He was admitted to the clinic and treated with parenteral penicillin. The hemorrhoids were in fact condyloma lata and appropriate stains revealed the presence of treponema pallidum in them.

In the early 80s, several young men presented for evaluation of lumps in the neck. Extensive tests including biopsy of these large lymph nodes were non-revealing. Later on in that decade

---

[78] *Hemorrhoidectomy*: The surgical removal of hemorroids, which are dilated veins in the anal canal and rectum.

[79] *Silver Stain*: A stain that colors the spirochetes of syphilis, among other things, to help the organisms stand out under the microscope.

[80] *Spirochetes*: Spiral-shaped bacteria that are found in patients with syphilis.

[81] *Syphilis*: A disease transmitted through sexual contact due to an organism called treponema pallidum. It may cause what looks like hemorrhoids, but they are in fact condylomata lata, which are growths around the anal opening seen in secondary syphilis.

HIV (human immune-deficiency virus) was detected in homosexual men. This virus was discovered to be transmitted mainly in men having sex with men already infected with the HIV. This virus diminishes the ability of the body to resist dealing with infections by decreasing the number of CD4[82] cells. Extensive research has resulted in the discovery and use of antiviral agents which can keep the virus suppressed and allow the HIV-infected patients to live a reasonable life. Before the introduction of these antiviral drugs, HIV patients were prone to a variety of diseases some of which were fatal.

I recall having to admit a middle-aged man who presented with malaise, fever, and a cough associated with shortness of breath. A chest X-ray showed multiple patchy infiltrates of unclear aetiology[83]. Dr. Robert Sarnoff of the Pulmonary Division carried out a bronchoscopy and a lung biopsy. This revealed the presence of pneumocystis carinii[84] to which HIV patients are prone to. A little while later, the patient developed encephalomyelitis[85] with lower limb paralysis. An extensive

---

[82] *CD4:* The name given to lymphocytes which have the ability to kill the HIV virus. The lower the CD4 cells, the more prone one is to the complications of HIV.

[83] *Aetiology*: Cause.

[84] *Pneumocystis carinii:* The organism that causes pneumonia in HIV patients.

[85] *Encephalomyelitis:* Inflammation of the brain and the spinal cord.

herpes genitalis eruption followed, the rash covering most of his back. These events took place prior to the availability of specific HIV drugs and the patient passed away.

Chapter 8

Uncharted Territory

~

"Providing Care with Limited Resources"

During my time at the clinic (1979 - 1986), work stress and the health crisis at home which went from bad to worse, I had a welcome visit from my brother Reza and his Iranian wife Fereshteh. Following extensive thought and discussion, it was decided (rightly, or otherwise) that I would move to the UK with my son Martin and start life anew. We found the family environment of my brother a relief and attempted to enter the medical market by setting up a cardiac evaluation clinic in Harley Street entitled "The Capital Diagnostic Center." We carried out physician evaluations by performing complete physical examinations and, when indicated, exercised stress testing with a cardiologist standing by. If necessary, echocardiography[86] was performed and interpreted by an expert

---

[86] *Echocardiography:* A machine that is moved up and down over the left side of the chest, sending waves to the heart. It receives the rebounding of these waves from the heart to the machine. These waves will tell you the status of the heart.

in that field. We had a soundproof room where hearing tests were done by an expert technician. We also had access to the London Clinic for routine laboratory testing and X-rays.

I myself saw patients when the opportunity arose and evaluated some cases of medical interest. These included diagnosing asymptomatic diabetes mellitus[87] in my sibling, finding severe aortic regurgitation with heart failure in a young man who had had a pig valve inserted 15-years prior to his visit for rheumatic aortic valve disease (the pig valve was successfully replaced by a cardiac surgeon at a nearby hospital), and a case of scleroderma[88] with widespread lung fibrosis but surprisingly no dyspnoea (shortness of breath) in an elderly lady for which no therapy was available.

For about a year and a half, we attempted to increase our patient flow by arranging lectures for the medical community and encouraging patient referrals without significant success. Ultimately, the Center was closed down. As luck would have it, it was at this time that a letter arrived from Dr. Hollingsworth inviting me to return to San Diego to join the Veterans

---

[87] *Asymptomatic diabetes mellitus:* A case of diabetes that is unknown to the patient. The diagnosis is made by testing the blood for its sugar level, which is abnormally high. The urine also contains sugar.

[88] *Scleroderma:* A condition where fibrous tissue involves the whole body. The skin becomes thick and tight, because of the excessive fibrous tissue in it.

Administration (VA) Medical Facility as a Professor of Medicine at UCSD (University of California, San Diego) and Head of the Division of General Internal Medicine. He envisioned an increase in the number of physicians providing care in the VA's Urgent Care Center and effectively running the outpatient clinics as outpatient centers were being planned and in the process of being constructed.

I accepted the position with enthusiasm and after getting married (the traditional Iranian way) to Fariba, a Persian lady of the illustrious Majd family on a trip to Tehran in 1990, I returned to San Diego, purchased a condominium, and proceeded on my venture of building up a large and impressive department of General Internists providing outstanding care to our veterans as well as supervising and teaching the medical school's house officers and medical students.

Within a year of my arrival in San Diego, we were delighted to be blessed by the arrival of a beautiful girl we named Lillygol June. Three years later, we were elated to add a second daughter to the family whom we named Lara Laadan. She seemed to be prone to asthma, which cleared up with the passage of time, requiring a single night's stay at the San Diego Children's Hospital.

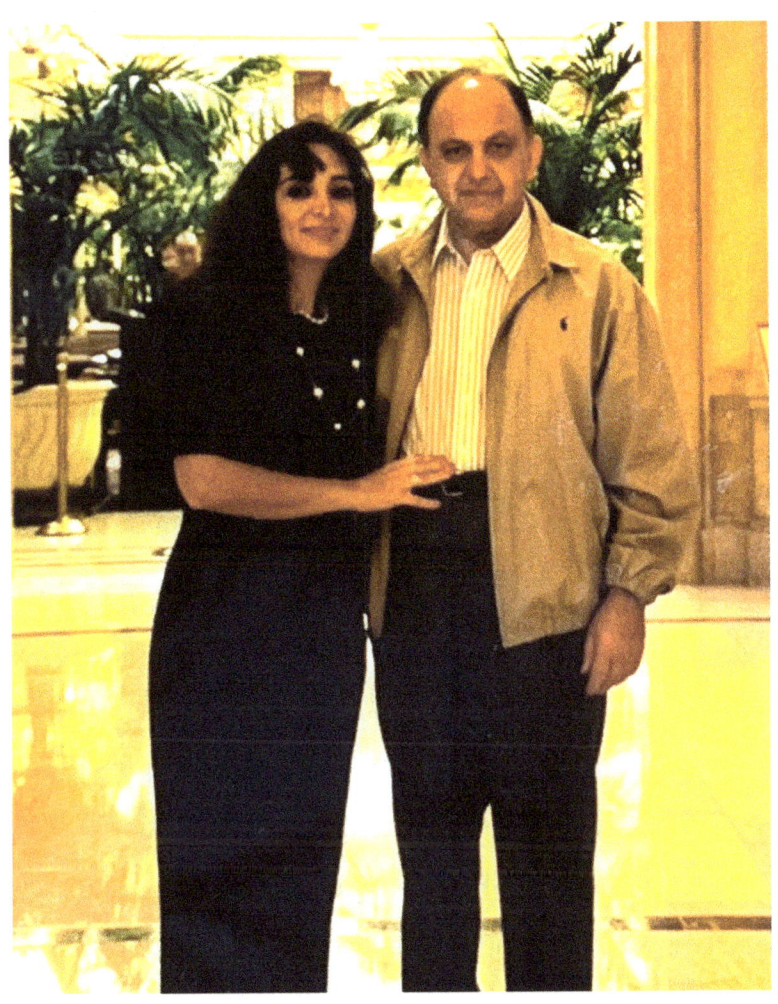

Fariba and me at the Bellagio Hotel in Las Vegas.

It was about this time that my Chief Dr. William Hollingsworth decided to retire. His replacement was Dr. Roger Spragg, who was a pulmonologist and more of a researcher than a clinician. It became quite clear to me that he really wanted a researcher with multiple grants rather than a clinician to lead the Division of

General Internal Medicine. We had conflicting plans on how to expand and organize the section with him wanting a researcher to do the job. He had several candidates in mind, none of whom were interested in the position.

When I first arrived at the VA Medical Center in San Diego to create a section of General Medicine and Geriatrics, I was provided with a small room in the Neurology Department. At that time, there were a handful of physicians running the urgent care center and several physicians seeing patients at the Mission Valley Clinic.

I met with Dr. Spragg on multiple occasions, pointing out the need for additional providers, space, particularly at the VA Site and secretarial assistance. He didn't seem too concerned about my requests and in fact made little effort to respond to my correspondence.

I stayed on as Chief of the Section, increasing the faculty from 5 to 40 physicians. There were several reasons for the enthusiasm of physicians in joining the Section of General Internal Medicine and Geriatrics (GIMG). These included the provision of time to evaluate patients (an hour for a new case and a half-hour for a revisit), protected time for research (half a day per week), an increase in salary, sufficient time for continuing medical education (grand rounds, daily morning conferences, and the opportunity to teach medical students and house staff). The substantial increase in applications to join our section allowed us to handpick outstanding candidates for available positions. Within a few years, the Section of GIMG became the largest in the UCSD Department of Medicine.

The section at the VA was part of the UCSD Division of GIMG. I had monthly meetings to update Dr. J. Ramsdale, the Division Chief of the VA section's activities, recruitments, teaching, research activities, and patient care.

It is difficult to praise any single physician in our Section for outstanding work ethic but praise must be bestowed on all members for their dedication and hard work in making the Section second to none in the country.

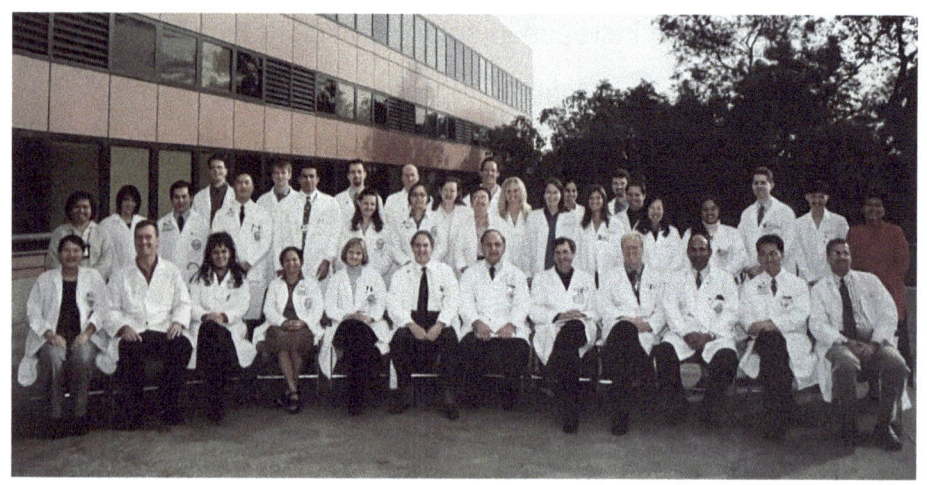

Members of the Division of General Internal Medicine at the VA in 2004. I am seated in the middle of the front row with Dr. Gass on my right and Dr. Kaushansky, Chair Department of Medicine at UCSD School of Medicine, on my left. Dr. Hilda Thorisdottir is on Dr. Gass's right, and Dr. Manju Woytowitz is third from the left in the front row. Dr. Bradj Pandey is seated third from the right in the front row, and Dr. Tuan Dang is on Dr. Pandey's left.

For this, in April 2005, I was awarded the VA's Leadership Award, where I was cited as *"an exceptional leader in the general internal medicine section… an outstanding mentor for the junior faculty. His love for furthering medical education is well known. He was instrumental in instituting a bi-weekly, one-hour educational conference for the attending physicians. He also runs a morning lecture series for the house-staff and medical students on a daily basis. Both lecture series qualified for CMA (Continuing Medical Education) credit. For these accomplishments, he is recognized with the Excellence in Leadership award."*

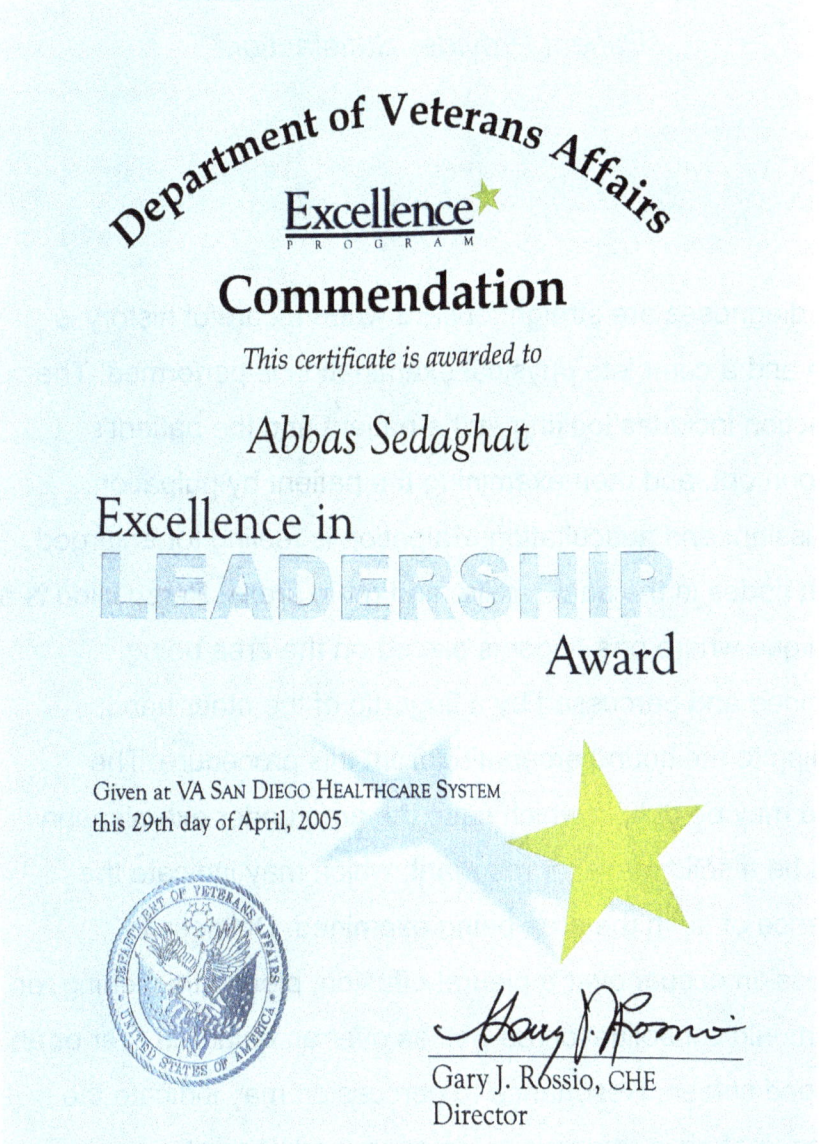

Chapter 9

Persistence Pays Off

~

"Patient Provider Satisfaction"

Most diagnoses are straightforward when a careful history is taken and a complete physical examination is performed. The inspection includes looking at the patient and the patient's environment, and then examining the patient by palpation, percussion, and auscultation. Palpation is feeling for enlarged lymph nodes in the neck, axilla, and groin areas. Percussion is a technique where one finger is placed on the area being examined and percussed by a fingertip of the other hand, listening to the sound emanating from this procedure. The sound may be dull, in which case the area under examination could be a solid mass, or resonant, which may indicate the presence of air in the area being examined. Dullness to percussion occurs over a pleural effusion, pleural thickening, or pneumonic consolidation as well as over an enlarged liver or an enlarged spleen. Resonance to percussion may indicate the presence of air in the area being examined; for instance, it might indicate a collapsed lung, as in cases of pneumothorax. This is followed by auscultation, where one listens with the stethoscope to the heart, lungs, and abdomen for any abnormal sounds. Well-trained physicians consider the differential diagnosis as they proceed with the examination. Kyphoscoliosis[89] is easily detected on observation of the spine and may be associated with compromised lung function. Tactile fremitus[90] may be absent in pneumothorax[91], pleural thickening of asbestosis[92] as well as a pleural effusion.[93] Auscultation[94] may reveal bronchial breathing[95] of consolidation, pleural rub of pleuritis[96] and be absent on the left side in endotracheal intubation when the tube has descended into the right main bronchus. Wheezing is

---

[89] *Kyphoscoliosis:* when the spine is bent forward and laterally.

[90] *Tactile fremitus:* vibration one feels when the hand is put on the chest and the patient is asked to say a sentence.

[91] *Pneumothorax:* when the lung collapses and there is air between the collapsed lung and the wall of the chest.

[92] *Pleural thickening of asbestosis:* the tissue that covers the lung (pleura), and a similar layer covering the inside of the chest wall may be thickened by asbestosis. The two layers are separated from each other, which may be due to the presence of air or fluid between the lung and the chest wall.

[93] *Pleural effusion:* when there is fluid in the pleural space.

[94] *Auscultation:* when one listens to the lung sounds with a stethoscope.

[95] *Bronchial breathing*: a reverse in normal breathing pattern. In a normal patient, the lung sounds follow prolonged inspiration and short expiration. In bronchial breathing, one hears a long expiration and a short inspiration.

[96] *Pleural Rub of Pleuritis:* when there is inflammation of the pleura (covering the lung and the chest wall). If one breathes deeply, one may hear the two walls of the pleura rubbing against each other.

audible in asthma and acute exacerbations of COPD[97] and/or a foreign body in the airway in children playing with toys of the appropriate size.

The need to speed up the physical examination because of time constraints has resulted in the lung and abdominal exams being performed perfunctorily with the patient being fully clothed! This has resulted in reliance on radiographic findings as a substitute for a productive physical examination of the body. There has been a complete disappearance of the neurological exam by physicians in a hurry to see as many patients as possible to generate income and to leave time for putting in the data in the electronic medical record. The computerization of medicine speeds up access to previous data on the patient being evaluated at the cost of mistakes being made by the physician in a hurry to get on with the next case. Many patients are unhappy that the physician is not looking at or listening to them as they seem to be focusing on data in the computer.

My approach is to teach the students to listen with care to the patient's history, proceed with a careful and complete physical examination followed by consideration of the differential diagnosis. Appropriate and relevant tests should be arranged, and the results should be discussed with empathy with the

---

[97] COPD: Chronic Obstructive Pulmonary Disease that cigarette smokers develop because of excessive smoking.

concerned patient. Third and fourth year students are taught how to elicit patient findings and then to go about presenting the case in a concise and relevant manner. Many cases of interest present at UCSD and the VA Medical Center's Urgent Care Center. I make a point of seeing each patient myself, gathering the medical students and the house staff in the examination room, and pointing out any significant findings in the case. This is followed by a discussion of the differential diagnosis and making arrangements for patient tests (if necessary), treatment, and follow-up. The students are encouraged to read the literature about cases we had seen together. Some of these cases were presented at our daily morning conferences and weekly M&M sessions. I made an effort to get specialists at the Medical Center to attend some of these meetings.

Every year, all medical students were required to vote for the attending staff who had inspired and taught them the most. In June 1993, I was surprised and delighted to be awarded a certificate at the UCSD Graduation Ceremony, which had the following notation on it, "University of California, San Diego School of Medicine June 1993 The Kaiser Permanente Award for Excellence in Teaching Presented by the Senior Class of the School of Medicine to Dr. Abbas Sedaghat with Deep Gratitude and Appreciation for his Continued Dedication to Teaching."

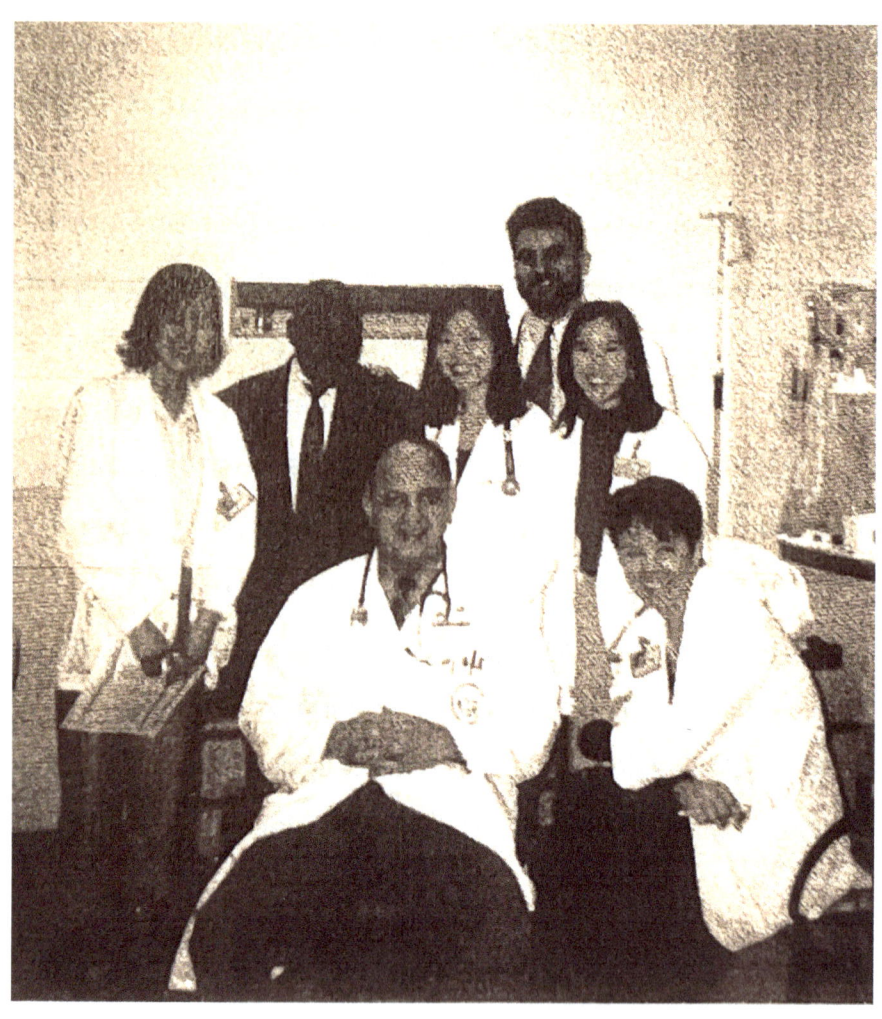

Surrounded by fourth year UCSD medical students in one of the VA Medical Center's Urgent Care Center examination rooms, 1995.

In 1996, I was delighted with a Teaching Award from the Junior Students. These were third year students whom I met every Monday afternoon for two hours, seeing and discussing cases of interest. Prior to these meetings, I would go on the wards and handpick patients suitable for presentation to the Junior students.

All in all, I was presented with 10 Teaching Awards by the Senior Students and 7 Awards by the Junior Students. The Medical School rules were that a consultant with 10 awards was no longer eligible for further accolades. After the graduation ceremony, which included a distinguished out-of-town speaker, tea was served, at which time I mingled with my students and their families, congratulating them and having photographs taken with them. That evening, a dinner party was held in honor of the graduates. Multiple speakers had their say and a memorable time was had by all.

July 28, 1999

MEMO TO: Abbas Sedaghat, M.D.
Clinical Professor

SUBJECT: Congratulations

Dear Abbas,

I wish to congratulate you, once again, on your receipt of the Kaiser Award for Excellence in Teaching for the seventh year in a row.

Stephen I. Wasserman, M.D.
The Helen M. Ranney Professor and
Chairman, Department of Medicine

UNIVERSITY OF CALIFORNIA, SAN DIEGO

BERKELEY • DAVIS • IRVINE • LOS ANGELES • RIVERSIDE • SAN DIEGO • SAN FRANCISCO 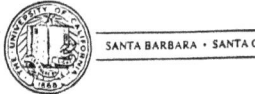 SANTA BARBARA • SANTA CRUZ

OFFICE OF THE DEAN
SCHOOL OF MEDICINE
June 1, 1999

9500 GILMAN DRIVE
LA JOLLA, CALIFORNIA 92093-0602

Abbas Sedaghat, M.D.
Clinical Professor, Department of Medicine (9111)

Dear Dr. Sedaghat:

Once again, it with considerable pleasure that I write to inform you that you have been chosen by the students to receive the Kaiser Award for Excellence in Teaching. Again this year, both the Senior Class and the Junior Class selected you as the outstanding faculty member. As you know, recipients are selected by a vote of the student body and awards are announced officially at Commencement ceremonies.

I hope very much that you will be able to arrange your schedule to participate in the event on Sunday, June 6, if you have not already planned to do so.

On behalf of the School, let me take this opportunity to extend congratulations and express the hope that you will continue your valuable contributions in the critical area of teaching.

With best regards.

Sincerely,

John F. Alksne, M.D.
Vice Chancellor for Health Sciences
Dean, School of Medicine

c: Dr. S. Wasserman (8811-W)

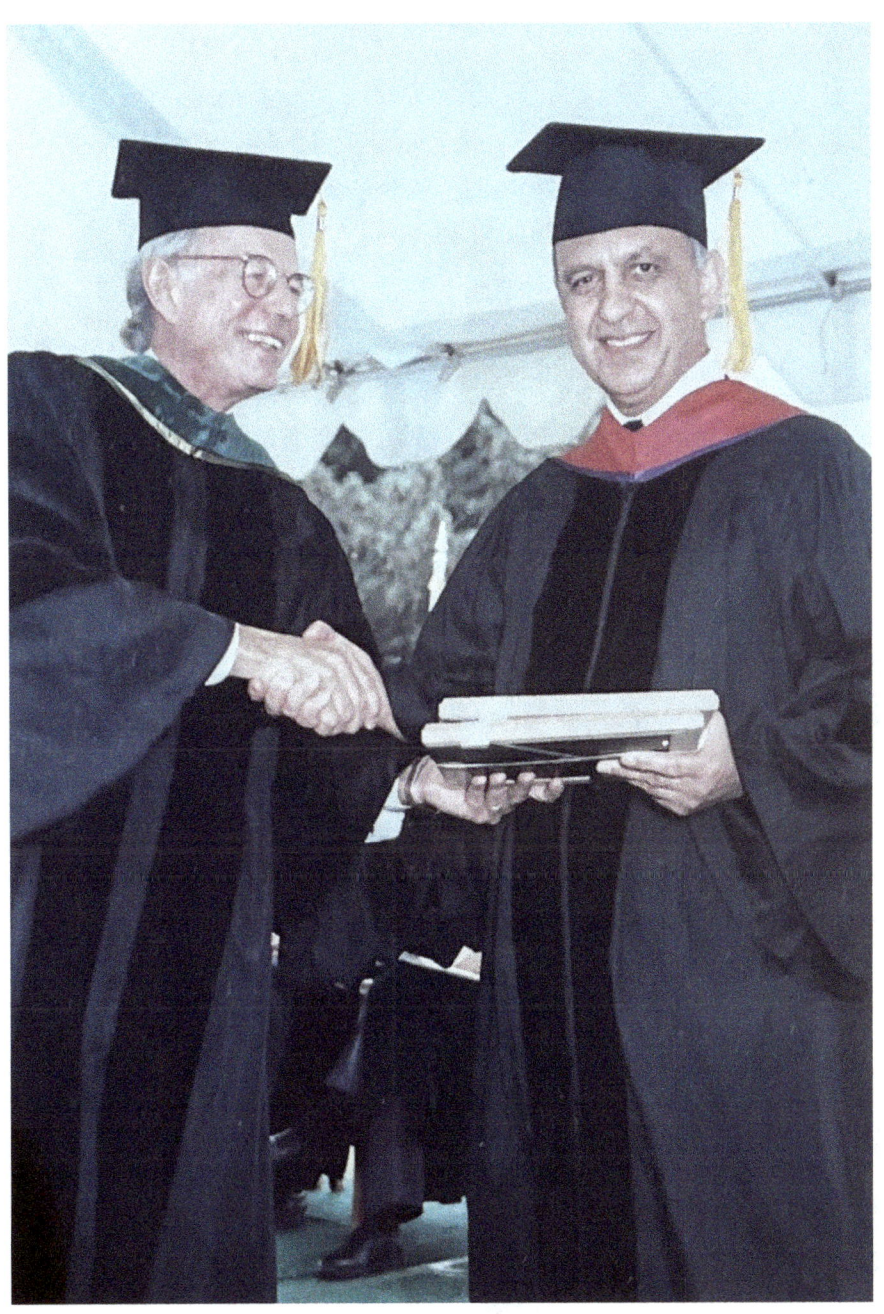

The Dean of the UCSD Medical School presenting me with two teaching awards, 1996.

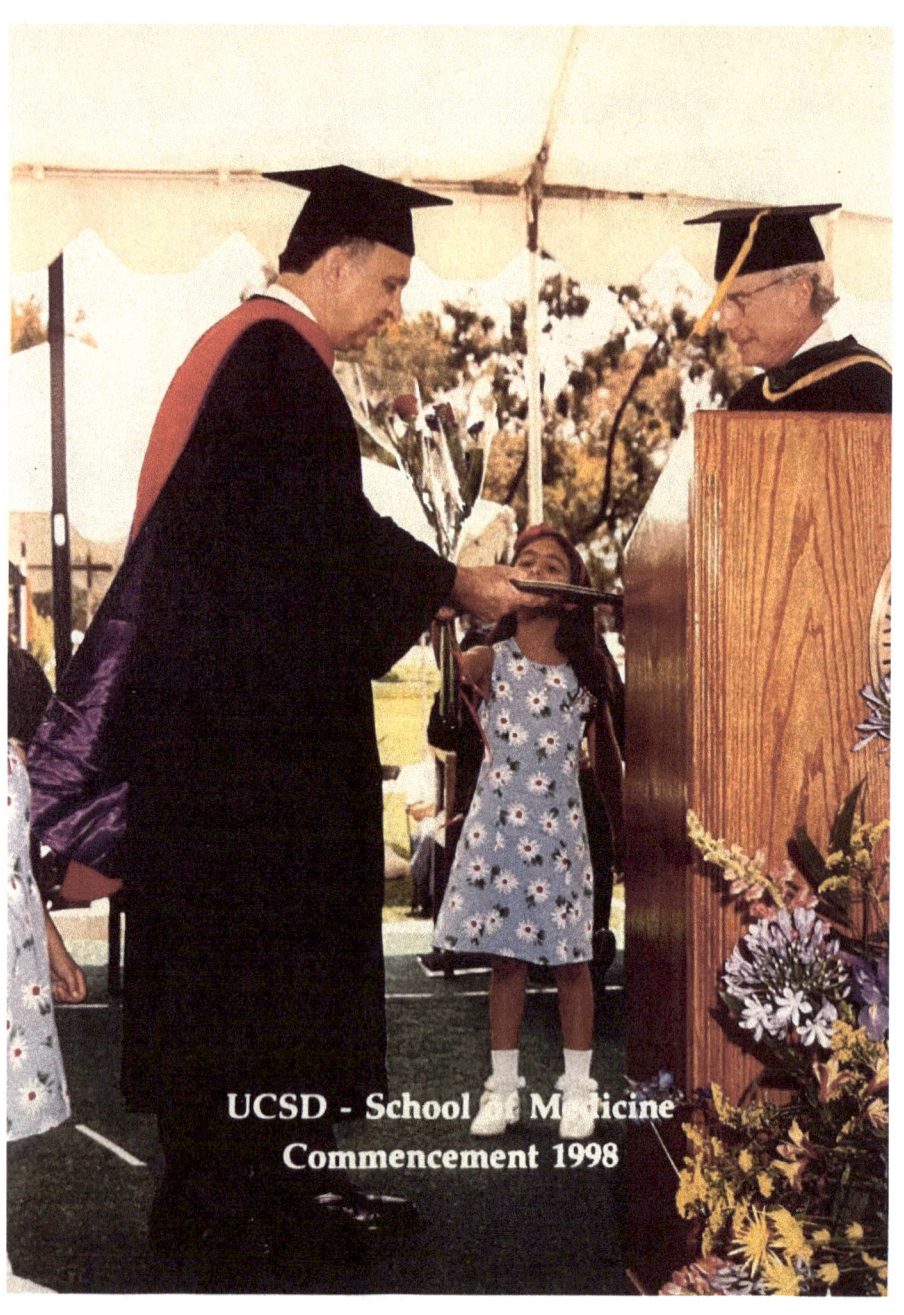

One of the many teaching awards presented to me by the Dean of UCSD School of Medicine in 1998.

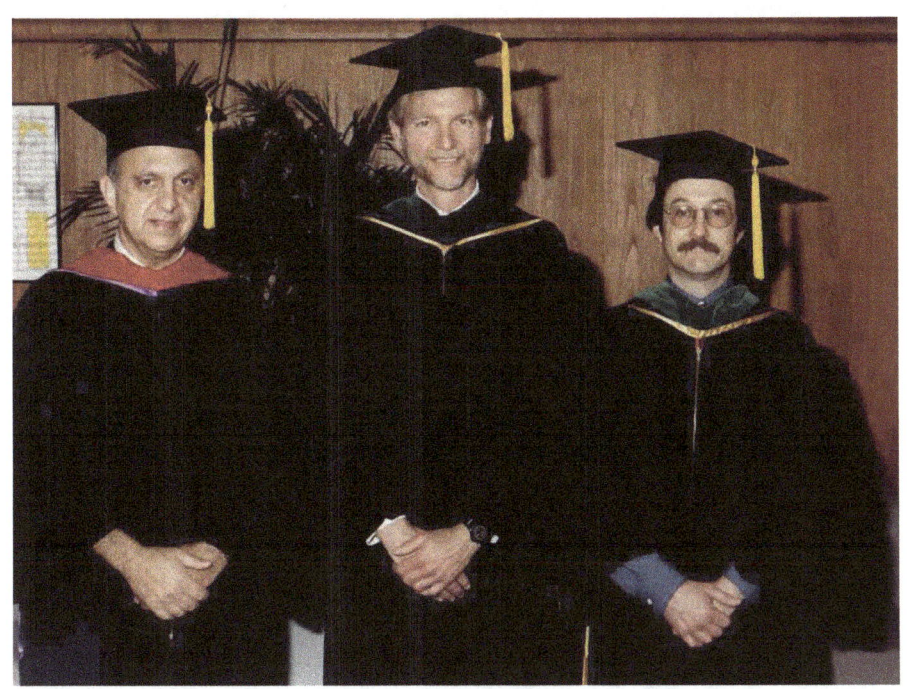

Teaching awards in the early 2000 to me (on the left) from the Junior and Senior Students; the Teaching Award winner from the second year students to Dr. L. Hansen (in the middle), and the first year students award winner Dr. M. Kritchevsky (on the right).

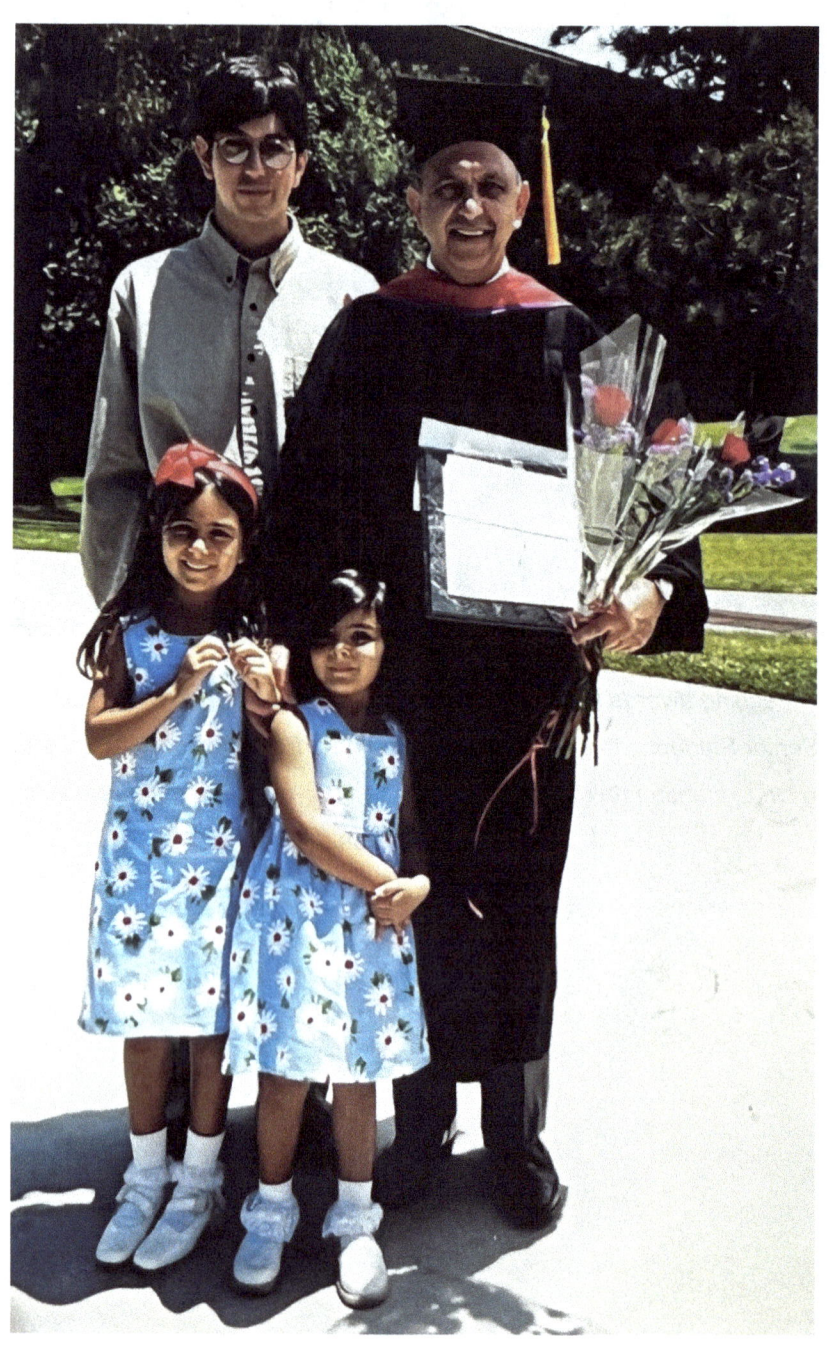

Martin, Lilly, and Lara with me on Graduation Day in 1998.

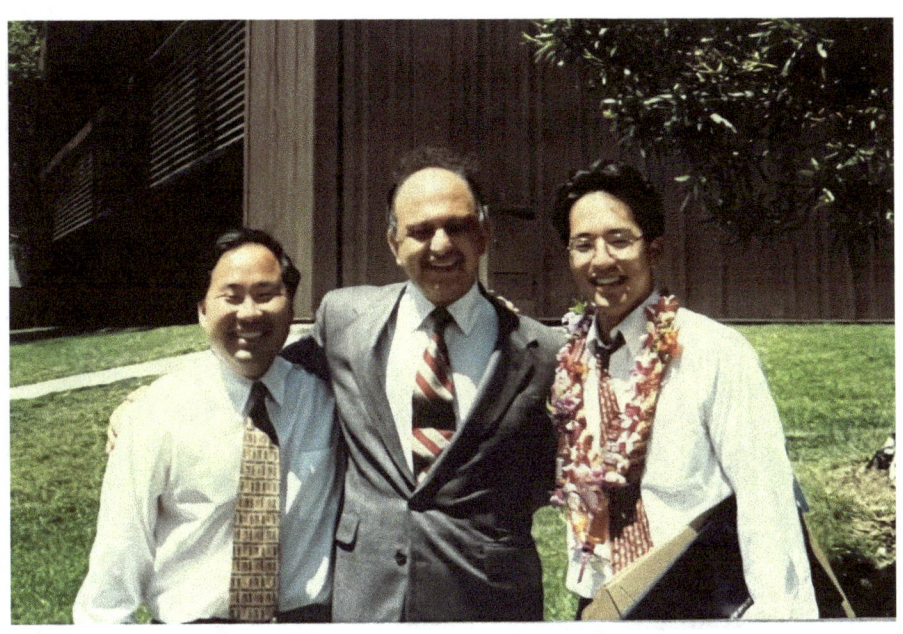

With two of my graduating fourth-year students.

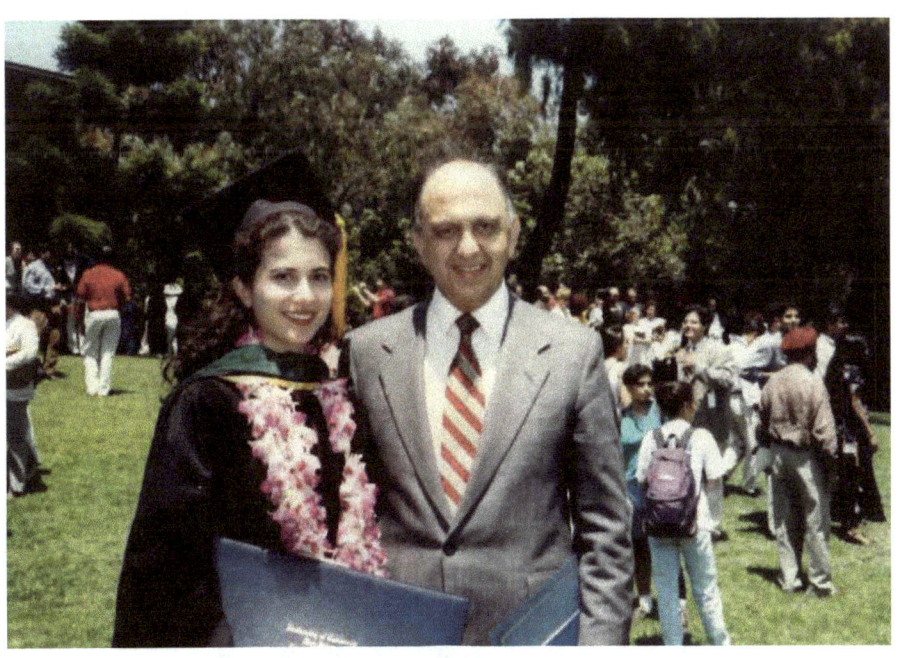

One of my Iranian students at the graduation ceremony.

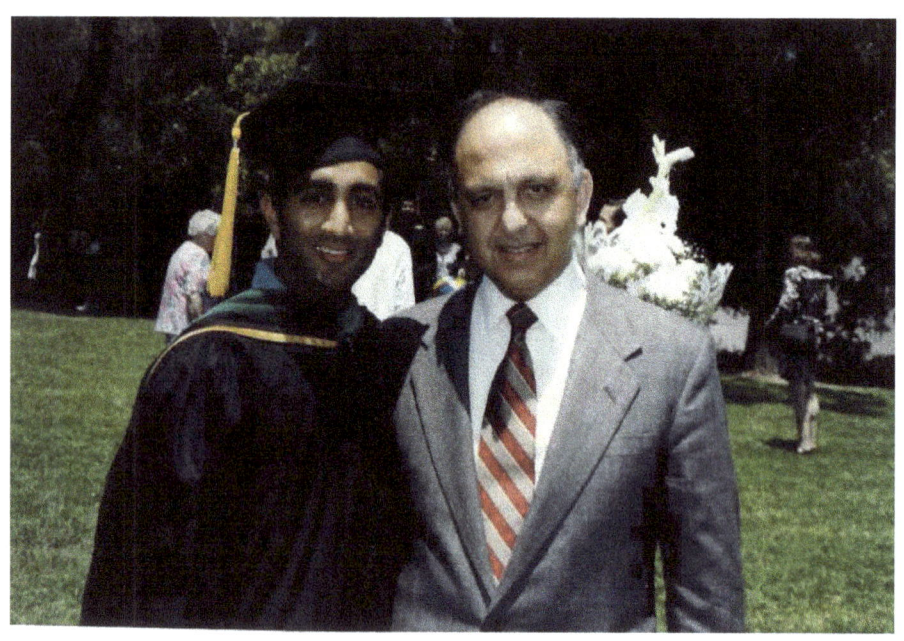

The graduation of another of my students at UCSD.

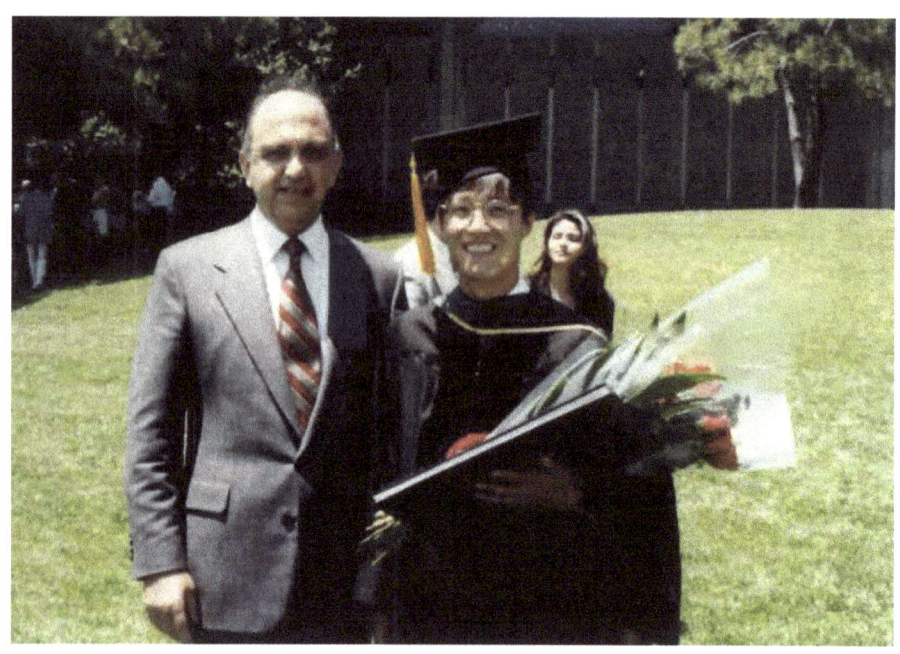

Another happy fourth-year student on graduation day at UCSD.

The Senior students enjoyed their Urgent Care Center (UCC) rotation. We saw many cases of interest, diagnosed them following relevant tests, and then had the cases presented at our morning report sessions. Some of the diagnoses were made by careful observation of the patients on entering their rooms.

These "spot diagnoses" included acromegaly[98], rheumatoid arthritis[99], acute closed angle glaucoma[100], atheroembolism[101], DJD (degenerative joint disease)[102], COPD (chronic obstructive pulmonary disease), asthma as well as ascites[103] secondary to liver cirrhosis.[104] Following certain tests, we diagnosed many

---

[98] *Acromegaly:* excessive production of growth hormone by the pituitary gland, resulting in an enlargement of the body in general, including enlarged hands and feet, prominent jaw, and prominence of the supraorbital ridges (at the eyebrow areas).

[00] *Rheumatoid Arthritis:* an autoimmune disease where there is swelling of the body's joints associated with increased warmth and pain of the joints affected.

[100] *Acute closed angle glaucoma:* this presents with pain in the affected eye, mid-dilation of the pupil, and excessive increase in the eye's intraocular pressure.

[101] *Atheroembolism:* embolism of atheromatous material (cholesterol deposits on the inside of arteries) following arterial catheterization.

[102] DJD: arthritis, when the cartilage that covers the bony components of a joint degenerates. The joint becomes swollen and painful.

[103] *Ascites:* The presence of excessive fluid in the abdominal cavity usually due to liver cirrhosis.

[104] *Liver cirrhosis:* when excessive alcohol consumption results in excessive scar tissue in the liver, resulting in accumulation of fluid in the peritoneal cavity (the space in the abdomen between the liver and the spleen, the small and large bowel).

cases of ischemic heart disease[105], a patient with aortic dissection[106], one with IgA nephropathy[107], many cases of diabetes mellitus[108], some with major complications including peripheral neuropathy[109], retinopathy[110], arthropathy[111], nephropathy[112], and peripheral vascular disease[113]. Ascites usually due to alcoholic liver disease was a common finding.

---

[105] *Ischemic heart disease:* the heart getting insufficient blood supply due to cholesterol-containing material called atheromatous plaques which are deposited in the blood vessels leading to the heart, diminishing its blood supply. The heart doesn't function properly because it doesn't get sufficient blood.

[106] *Aortic dissection:* instead of the heart getting the blood supply through the whole of the artery, it goes through a part of the artery, because there is an opening in the inside of the blood vessel, causing blood to flow in the dissection of the wall of the artery. This decreases the space in which blood can flow to the artery and supply it with nutrients.

[107] *IgA Nephropathy*: a kidney disease, where a protein (IgA, which stands for immunoglobulin) causes damage to the kidney. In the blood, if there is more IgA than normal, it interferes with function of the kidney and doesn't allow it to operate properly.

[108] *Diabetes Mellitus:* an increase in sugar in the blood.

[109] *Peripheral neuropathy:* when the blood sugar is high, it may cause nerve damage, which means a patient gets numbness in the fingers, toes, etc. caused by damage to the nerves that serve those areas.

[110] *Retinopathy:* high blood sugar may cause damage to the lining of the eye, which causes a variety of patients with diabetes to have blindness.

[111] *Arthropathy:* damage to the joints of the body because of high blood sugar.

[112] *Nephropathy*: damage to the kidneys.

[113] *Peripheral Vascular Disease:* when there is a major block to the arteries supplying blood to the legs or the arms. It occurs in diabetic patients. The vessels are covered on the inside with atheromatous lesions containing cholesterol, which cut off the blood supply to the legs. Some patients may need to have an amputation.

Many physicians were interviewed for jobs at the now well-known VA Medical Center; the best of these were added onto the growing number of physicians working at that Institution. During the interview, I would observe their knowledge of English, their mode of dress, their reasons to want to become a physician, the colleges they had been to, and why they had chosen UCSD Medical Center to apply to. Many applicants showed their disappointment at being turned down and some even threatened legal action for discrimination. Only top applicants were considered worthy of being sent to the Chief of the Medicine Service for further consideration of joining the section.

One of the applicants to join our section at the Veterans Affairs Medical Center in 1992 was an accomplished internist, Dr. Bradj Pandey. Dr. Pandey had carried out his medical training in Calcutta, India, and his internal medicine residency in New York City. He was an excellent physician, a superb teacher of clinical medicine, a dedicated father and husband, and a reliable friend. His charming wife Manjula and his two wonderful sons (Prashant and Amit) were supportive members of the family. I spent many memorable evenings at the Pandey residence enjoying Manjula's delicious cooking and our far-ranging discussions about current affairs, world history, medical practice, medical research, family issues, religion, etc. Dr. Pandey is now retired and enjoys playing golf and spending time with family and friends.

In 2004, I was elected by UCSD to become a member of the Academy of Clinician Scholars. The latter award was presented to a handful of outstanding clinician scholars who had been of significant service to the medical center.

-----Original Message-----
From: Seakp@aol.com [mailto:Seakp@aol.com]
Sent: Thursday, March 11, 2004 6:15 PM
To: abbas.sedaghat@med.va.gov; mpian@ucsd.edu
Subject: Academy of Clinician Scholars

As President of the UCSD Academy of Clinician Scholars, I have the pleasure of informing you of your election into the Academy. You were nominated and elected by your clinical peers for outstanding clinical excellence, as well as contributions in teaching and scholarship. I apologize for the format of this notification, but with the next meeting of the Academy on March 23, I wanted to announce the election results quickly. Formal letters will be going out in a few days.

I am attaching a copy of the bylaws. Gene Hemmerling will be sending you an Academy roster with contact information.

More info on the meeting to follow.

Best Wishes,
Angela Scioscia

A letter informing my election to become a member of the Academy of Clinician Scholars.

Chapter 10

Progress on the Home Front

~

"From Berkeley to Japan with an Interlude in Oxford"

During my sixteen years as Chief of the General Internal Medicine - Geriatrics Section at the VA Medical Center, I participated in visiting Tehran and Shiraz one month per year as a visiting professor. I gave lectures, tutorials, acted as Ward Attending, and saw individual patients per request of the other attendings. On these occasions, I stayed with my gracious sister Gohar and her family when in Tehran.

During the four years as Professor of Medicine in Shiraz, I did some research and published several articles in the *Pahlavi Medical Journal*. These included articles on toxoplasmosis, cholera, subclinical infection with mycobacteria in southern Iran, malaria, management of acute barbiturate intoxication, and the status of tuberculin skin testing at the Pahlavi University Medical Center, now called the University of Shiraz (a result following the Iranian Revolution).

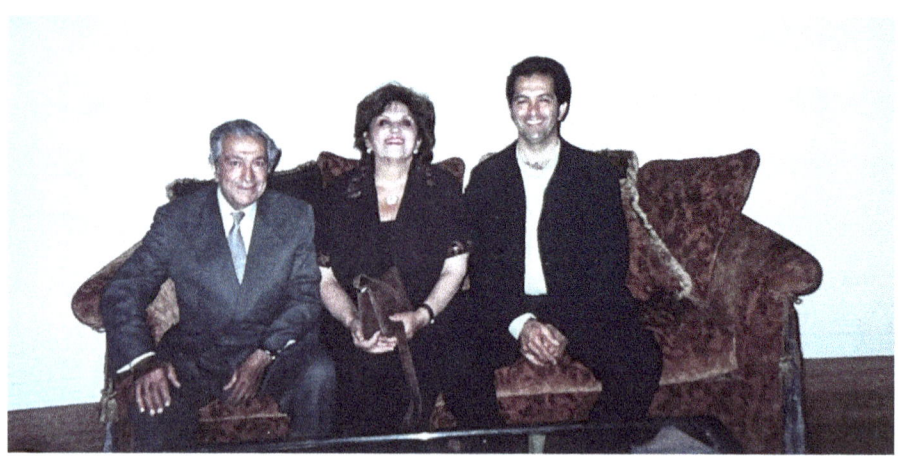

My sister in the family's splendid home in Tehran flanked by her husband, Dr. M. Matin (a fine OBGYN specialist) and their eldest son Kamran (a cardiologist in the Los Angeles area).

I was given a six-months sabbatical to go abroad and assess the teaching of clinical medicine to medical students and house staff in several medical centers. I visited the School of Medicine in Glasgow, Scotland and medical student teaching in several countries including the Karolinska Institute in Stockholm, Sweden, the Hammersmith Hospital as well as the Royal Free Hospital in London, England, and the Schools of Medicine in Tehran and Shiraz. A full report was compiled and sent to the senior individuals at the VA Medical Center as well as the UCSD School of Medicine. The only feedback I got was through an intermediary who stated that there was surprise and concern about the end of the report, where it was stated that recently graduated Iranian physicians could not find jobs and were found to carry out other activities such as driving taxis to be able to survive! Many of such physicians were eager to emigrate to find work in other countries. An article published in the *Annals of Internal Medicine* in 1971 by Dr. H. Ronaghy, a consultant physician at the Pahlavi University Medical Center (PUMC) found that 90% of Iranian MDs visiting the USA did not return to their own country.

Dr. H. Ronaghy, an astute and experienced clinician, had a different approach to healthcare in Iran in general and Shiraz, in particular. He and his hospitable wife Sima (also a physician) trained a substantial number of high school graduates in the City of Shiraz as well as in outlying areas (in the vicinity of a town called Kazeroon) in the basics of healthcare. Such persons were able to provide on the spot evaluation and treatment of sick individuals. Any complex cases were referred to the PUMC for expert assessment and therapy. This novel approach to healthcare was an excellent way to bypass the need for trained physicians in areas where they were needed but not attracted to live in.

Another fine physician I got to know and respect in Shiraz was the renowned head of the Department of Pathology at the

PUMC by the name of Professor Parviz Haghighi. He and his dedicated wife Parry, who practiced pediatrics, had two fine sons, one of whom became a dermatologist later in life. Parviz was a superb and highly dedicated pathologist. His services and opinions were in great demand in Shiraz, Iran and at UCSD as well as the VA Medical Center in San Diego, where he worked for many years training outstanding residents in that field.

During my sabbatical, Reza and I visited Kish Island just off the southern coast of Iran in the Persian Gulf, where Sadegh, my youngest brother, had set up a coffee importing and distribution center. His daughter, a bright young lady, was studying Computer Science at the local university. We spent several days in Kish Island enjoying the sunny weather, swimming and snorkeling.

My son Martin, an outstanding student and a gifted artist, was accepted by all UC colleges. He chose UC Berkeley, played badminton, kendo, and graduated in 2003. Then he headed for Japan as a participant in the JET program, where he taught English to Japanese students. He met Chigusa, a charming and accomplished Japanese psychologist. She spoke English perfectly and invited many of her friends to a superb wedding held at the famous Estancia Hotel in La Jolla, CA, enjoyed immensely by all present. The Reverend John Huber carried out the marriage ceremony, who, several years earlier, had baptized Martin. Because of Martin's enthusiasm, hard work, and ability, he became an excellent teacher of English and the Japanese authorities hung on to him as an accomplished, desirable, and responsible teacher.

A poem for my Dad,
By Martin Sedaghat

When times are tough
And life seems rough,
Though no one seems to care,
I hope you know that I am always there.

And when all and everything,
Seems to come to push and shove,
Remember that Christmas is a time to love.

Sometimes when you feel you're lost
And all you need comes at a cost,
Though you seem to live your life in fear,
Just remember all the good times,
And how much to me you're dear.

I Love You Daddy,
    Your Eternally Loving Son,
        Martin O X X X X X X X O

In 2012, the couple were blessed by the birth of a baby boy, who loves reading, skiing, tennis, rock climbing, and video games. He plays the piano and is working to master the abacus. He has a dog called Lupin, now 14 years of age, who protects the family by barking furiously when he hears the slightest sound. Martin is in the process of doing a Master's program online through the

University of Birmingham in the United Kingdom. He plans to become a university faculty member when he obtains his degree.

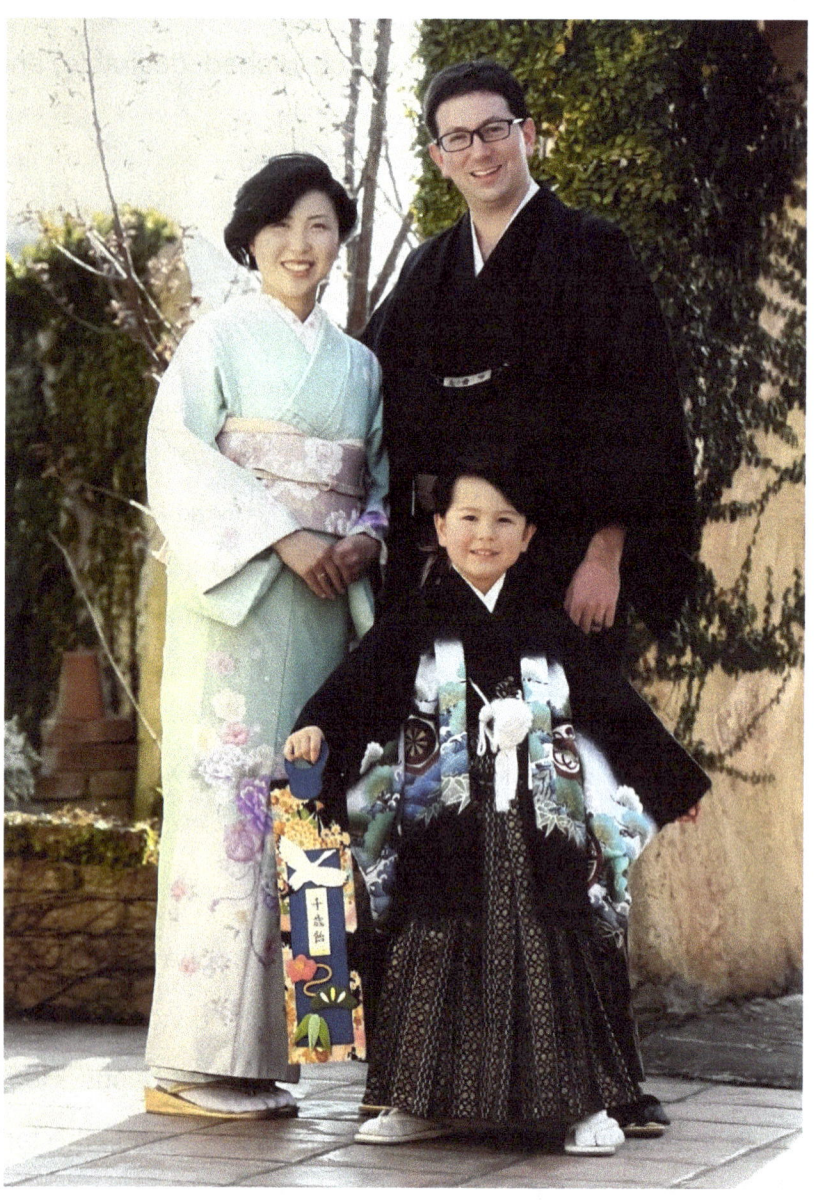

Martin, Chigusa, and their son, Allen in formal Japanese attire.

Lillygol, also a UC Berkeley graduate and a senior student speaker at the graduation ceremony, spent a year at the University of Oxford at St. Hilda's College in the United Kingdom, where she obtained her Master's degree in 2021. She is involved in saving the world from plastic and other forms of pollution. She has created several stories for the National Geographic Society on pollution in Taiwan, India, Bangladesh, and Egypt. She is a fine speaker and has the ability to involve important personalities in roundtable discussions on multiple pollution issues, such as through her work on the National Geographic Asia's podcast "Expedition: Earth."

Lara, also a graduate of UC Berkeley, has a special interest in helping incarcerated individuals to heal their trauma, obtain employment, and to also remain academically active. Through her Elevate You Foundation non-profit organization, she provides them with excellent CVs free of charge, keeps in touch with them by telephone and mail, and encourages them to read extensively so that they keep themselves informed of world affairs. Lara has written over one thousand letters, searching for jobs to help these unfortunate souls who have been kept away from society. She helped one of the incarcerated persons to publish a book on his involvement with gangs prior to being incarcerated. The book, "To Hell With a Gang" makes interesting reading. She has two handsome Doberman Pinschers who are dedicated to her and keep her company and protect her.

Recently, Lara started the production of beautiful candles, which are available to the public online, under the company name "Persian Garden." Lara works remotely with high school students and instructs them on how to complete their CVs and compose letters of application to colleges. She is an accomplished and highly organized individual with superior computer skills.

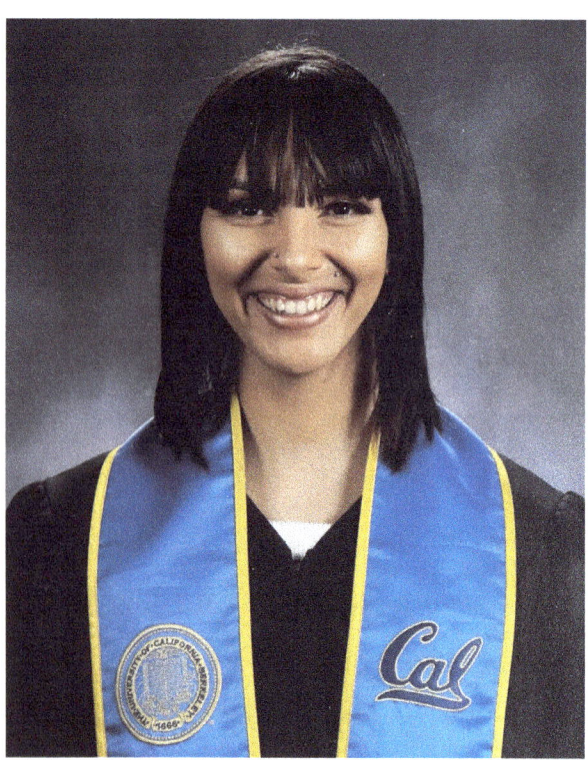

Lara at UC Berkeley graduation.

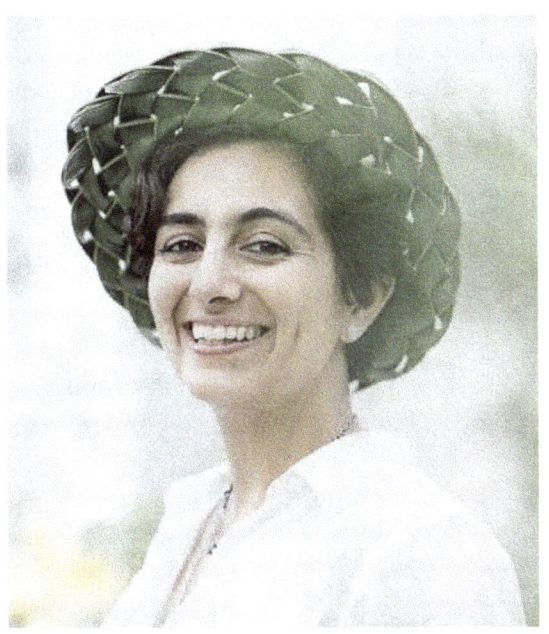

Lilly in Thailand happy at the end of her Ganges River Expedition, 2019.

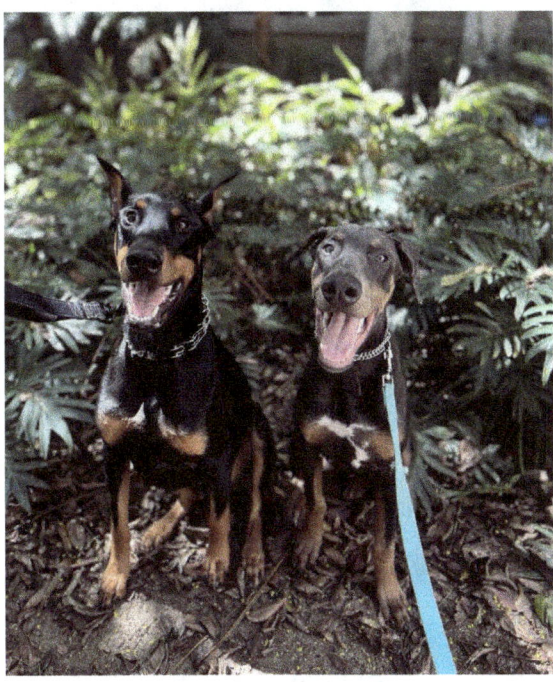

Lara's two Dobermans—Pharaoh on the left, Arctic on the right.

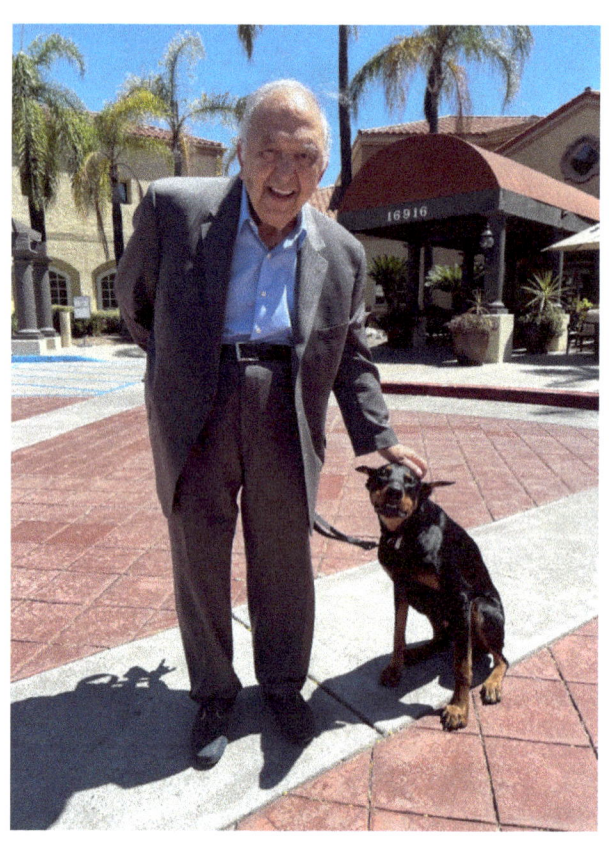

Me with Lara's oldest Doberman, Pharaoh.

In 2013, I made a trip to Japan to visit Martin and family. The cherry blossoms were in full bloom, looking absolutely gorgeous. During that visit, I got to take a look at the remains of Hiroshima following the American decision to use an atomic bomb to wipe out the city at the end of the Second World War. Very little remains of the target city, and it is a shame to have such places totally destroyed by these outrageous weapons!

On that same trip, I visited Lillygol in Beijing, where we took a bus to the Great Wall of China and visited the Forbidden City. Lilly took me on a walk to observe the food market and to horrify me by showing a variety of ants, cockroaches, scorpions, and starfish fried on a stick being consumed by hungry bystanders looking on.

After retiring from the VA Medical Center in 2006 at the age of 65, and feeling that I was still capable of being of service to society, I joined a group of physicians called the Home Physicians Medical Group created and run by a UCSD / VA colleague, Dr. Chris Hunt. I began working with this group in 2007, going to the home of patients needing medical care. The majority of such patients were covered by Medi-Care. Some were sick, requiring home visits; others were not ill and took advantage of the services provided by our group. A substantial number of these patients requested Norco for their back pain. I was not convinced that such patients needed home care and Norco and were abusing such medications to get high on them. One of the major issues was the lack of interest by Medi-Care and Medi-Cal in reimbursing physicians who were putting in time and effort for a large number of patients. This involved long periods of time, sometimes up to six months, to be remunerated for the work carried out.

In 2019, I accompanied Lillygol to London, where we were met by my brother Reza. He had made arrangements for us to go from Heathrow Airport directly to the city of Oxford. With winter approaching, the weather was becoming cold. We wore pullovers, scarves, and jackets of UC Berkeley and were frequently greeted by the statement, "Go Bears!" with those familiar with the American university system. And on one occasion, someone remarked, "Now that's a real school!"

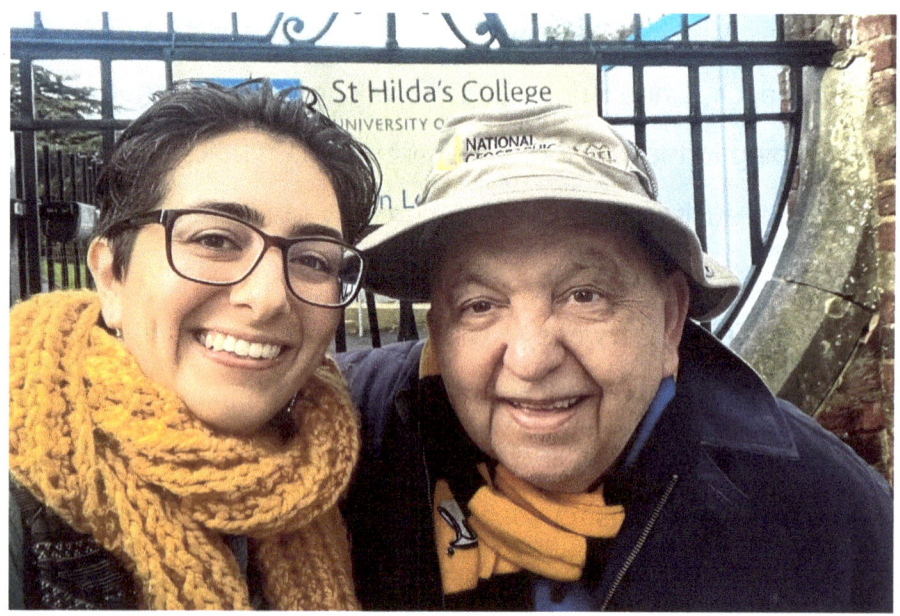

Lillygol and I pictured at Oxford University in front of St. Hilda's College in 2019.

During our ten-week stay in Oxford, we did a great deal of site-seeing, drank beer at several pubs (Lemonade Shandy specifically), and were impressed by the 40 colleges which formed the University of Oxford. Lilly's college (St. Hilda's) was initially an all-girls college, but now they allow male students to attend the college also. Lilly and I met with Dr. Ariell Ahearn, an American lady who was Course Director of the Nature, Society, and Environmental Governance Master's program at the School of Geography in Oxford. St. Hilda's College was one of the few all girls colleges which had had some success in the college rowing eights. It was situated in Cowley Place near the Magdalen Bridge. This was the site where a lot of courageous tourists had a go at the boats rowed by experts using poles to speed along the river under the Magdalen Bridge. These rivers joined each other to become the River Thames. The Botanical Gardens south of the Magdalen Bridge was a site to behold.

All colleges had a main gate quietly guarded by officially dressed porters who seemed to know all those coming in and out of the colleges and who were well-mannered and helpful. In fact, they allowed me to take the elevator to the Christ Church Dining Hall, instead of the stairs, both of which were featured in the popular Harry Potter films. Of interest to visitors was the Bridge of Sighs built in 1913, which joined the different parts of

Hartford College.

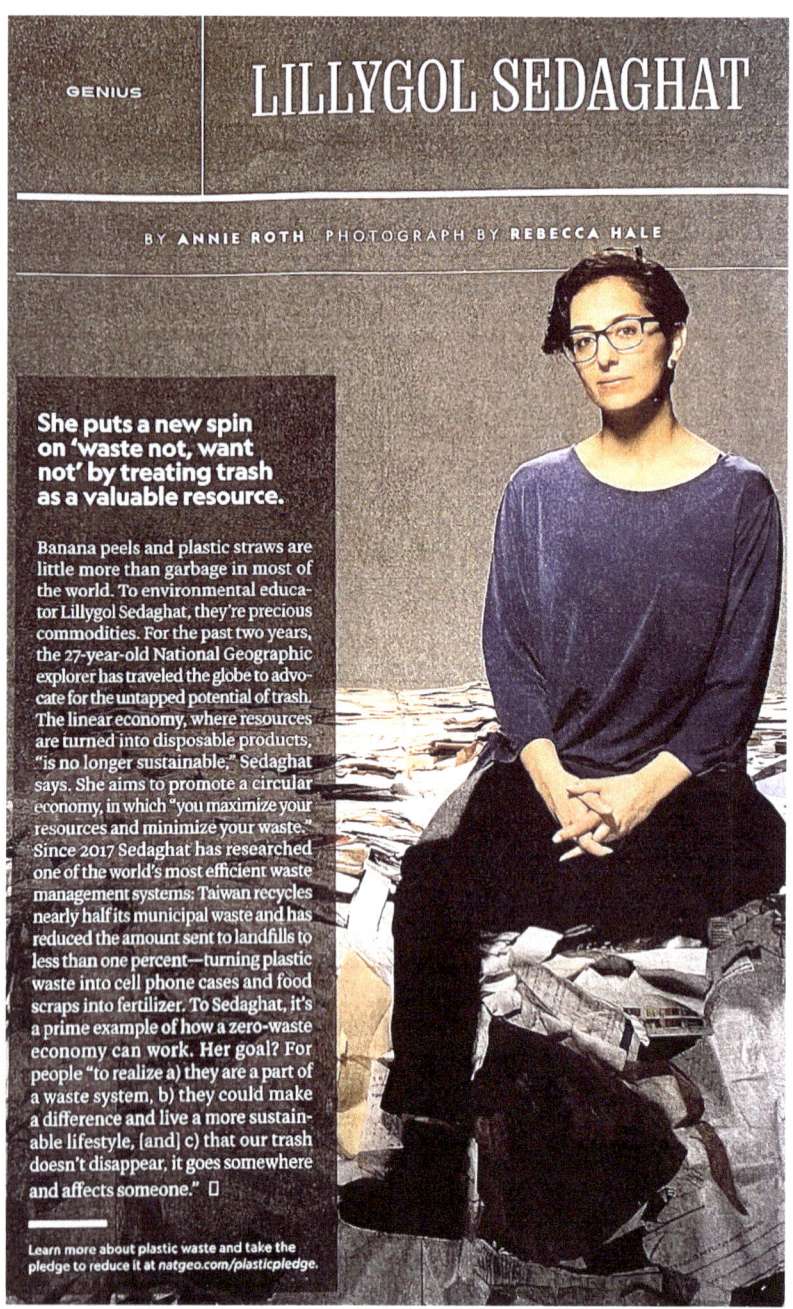

Lilly featured inside the National Geographic Magazine in December 2019.

Chapter 11

From Leeches to Heart Transplants: Lessons from the Medical Field

~

"The Beauty and the Beast"

Changes in the medical field, its practice, tests, treatments, and teaching have and continue to change. Most are beneficial for the patients, but some are detrimental as exemplified by the case I witnessed in the VA Medical Center where the Chief of Medicine developed angina.[114] An angiogram[115] was performed followed by coronary artery bypass surgery. The patient woke up with a severe right sided hemiplegia[116] presumably due to

---

[114] *Angina:* Pain in the chest on exertion, because of narrowing of the coronary arteries due to atherosclerosis.

[115] *Angiogram:* When a tube is put into an artery and passed all the way to the heart; dye is injected and pictures are taken that will show whether there is narrowing of the blood vessels that supply blood to the heart.

[116] *Hemiplegia:* When a part of the brain dies due to a lack of blood supply, resulting in a paralysis of half of the body. It is occlusion of blood vessels due to a variety of causes, the most common being atherosclerosis, which is a narrowing of the blood vessels due to cholesterol deposits.

atheroembolism during the operation. There has been little recovery of his condition over the years.

On call in the ER one evening at the VA Medical Center, a patient was sent from the cardiovascular unit having developed tender erythematous nodules on his legs. The diagnosis was straightforward; emboli of atheromatous plaques following angiography of the femoral arteries in a patient with intermittent claudication.

A disastrous case occurred when I was an attending physician in Shiraz, Iran. The wife of a colleague insisted on having abdominal liposuction. Post-surgery, she was and remains comatose. Lung infiltrates were seen in the chest X-ray and the brain MRI showed multiple areas of infarction[117] due to fat embolism[118]. The patient remains comatose to this day. My colleague sees patients during the day, and looks after his wife at night.

Telemedicine has become fashionable and is useful in situations where the physician is unable to examine the patient. In such

---

[117] *Infarction:* Death; In this case, an MRI of the brain showed patches of infarction of the brain tissue.

[118] *Fat embolism:* During liposuction, a needle is placed in the area to remove the fat; upon removal of the fat globules through aspiration, the fat globules can accidentally enter into the veins, go into the lungs, and cause lung damage, and end up in the brain, where they block the arterial supply and cause death of the brain tissue.

cases, a comprehensive history is available, but inspection is the only modality for examining the patient. Some disorders are easily diagnosable by observation alone and this mode of evaluation is of special value when the physician and patient are separated by significant distances and other obstacles. Having said that, it must be emphasized that there is no substitute for patient-physician face-to-face interaction, where palpation, percussion, and auscultation are available to the physician. Thus, the role of telemedicine is only of limited value at present.

To progress in this field, one has to study hard, see as many patients as possible, read journal articles as well as book chapters on the subject being studied, ask questions from teachers, discuss cases with friends, be polite to influential colleagues, and continue to learn throughout life.

In conclusion, the training and practice of medicine across the three continents can be summarized as follows:

United Kingdom - The boarding school experience resulted in lifelong friendships. Studying and playing sports in adverse environments such as being made to play rugby football on frozen pitches in winter resulted in being active in adverse environmental conditions. The scarce supply of food at meal times (initially being put down to rationing of the Second World War) kept the pupils thin, nimble, and fit.

The medical school system left much to be desired. The patient rounds were not particularly informative, were monotonous, but provided nursing input on the cases being discussed. The house officers were overworked, lacked sufficient sleep, and in particular, were only given the opportunity to attend a single grand rounds session per week, where they could learn something of substance. However, things are changing for the better! The house staff are given more time off duty, fewer nights on call, and are provided with more learning opportunities.

United States of America - The most significant finding was the time and effort put into teaching the house staff and medical students. This consisted of weekly ground rounds at which time a famous and knowledgeable physician or surgeon was invited to discuss a case or subject in depth. Everyday there were several lively sessions presented by members of the faculty at the Medical Center. Each morning at 7:00am, the house staff on call from the previous evening discussed any cases that had been admitted overnight. The students were dedicated and very keen to learn. I was invited to their homes on several occasions and enjoyed our discussions.

Iran - The standard of medical care in Shiraz was satisfactory, but there was room for improvement. Although it was considered to be one of the top medical schools in the country, having experienced the practice of medicine overseas, I was not overtly impressed by the type of medical care provided in that university city. In spite of the presence of a substantial number of the faculty having been trained in the US and Europe, the teaching of medicine to the students and house officers was considered to be far from ideal. My impression was that most of the medical students and house officers would prefer to be taught medicine in the US and UK. I was constantly harangued by senior medical students as well as house officers to facilitate their departure from Iran to Europe and America for continuing their studies and training.

This is not to belittle the house officers and attending staff for their efforts to teach the art of medical care to those attempting to promote their knowledge and ability in this most difficult field of human endeavors. There are many outstanding physicians and surgeons in Iran who have had excellent training overseas and who have returned to their country of birth to be of service to the large number of sick and ailing in the population. These include:

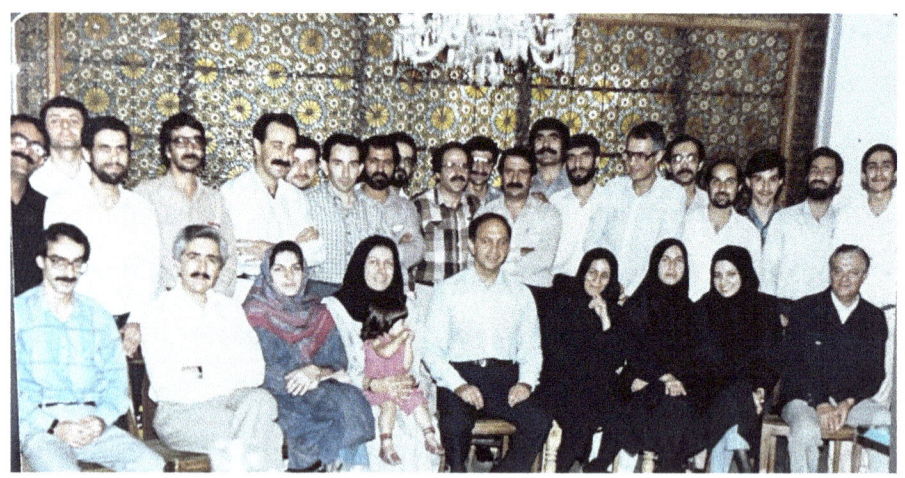

The attendings and house officers at the Medical Center in Shiraz, Iran.

- Dr. K. Nasr, who trained in gastroenterology at Columbia University School of Medicine in New York and was the Dean and force behind the creation of The Department of Medicine at the medical center in Shiraz, Iran.

- Dr. F. Ismail-Beygi, who was interested in disorders of the thyroid gland and was head of The Department of Medicine based at the Saadi Hospital.

- Dr. M. Sharmanesh, who trained at St. Thomas' Hospital Medical School in London and was an outstanding internist.

- Dr. Borhanmanesh, a gastroenterologist with a special interest in Hepatitis C.

- Dr. Haghshenas, a wonderful person who was an expert hematologist.

- Dr. Yeganehdoust, a pulmonologist.

- Dr. Hanjani, an accomplished cardiologist.

- Dr. Molavi, an expert infectious disease specialist.

- Dr. Rasregar, an exceptionally fine and knowledgeable nephrologist.

- Dr. Rejace, an excellent rheumatologist, who was very kind and dedicated and was my senior resident when I started work at Nemazee Hospital in 1974.

- Dr. Malekzadeh, who was one of my students in Shiraz and became the Minister of Health of the country. His main interest was gastroenterology and he was considered an authority on diseases of the liver. He was very kind to me and invited me to his home in Tehran on several occasions.

- Dr. Nasseri-Moghadam, who was second in command to Dr. Malakzadeh and was a delightful person. He was a generalist with a special interest in gastroenterology. On a trip to San Diego, he gave an excellent lecture at our grand rounds.

UCSD DEPARTMENT OF MEDICINE
GRAND ROUNDS

FEBRUARY 1999 — 8:30 A.M.

FEBRUARY 3
UCSD MEDICAL CENTER
MAIN AUDITORIUM

UPDATE ON LUNG CANCER
Wayne M. Saville, M.D., Assistant Adjunct Professor of Medicine
University of California San Diego

FEBRUARY 10
VA MEDICAL CENTER
MULTI-PURPOSE ROOM

WOMEN AND HEART DISEASE: WHY WE NEED CLINICAL TRIALS
Elizabeth Barrett-Connor, M.D., Professor of Family and Preventive Medicine
University of California San Diego

FEBRUARY 17
UCSD MEDICAL CENTER
MAIN AUDITORIUM

DEVELOPMENT OF GUIDELINES FOR THE DIAGNOSIS & TREATMENT OF ASTHMA
Harold Nelson, M.D., Professor of Medicine
University of Colorado Health Sciences Center

FEBRUARY 24
VA MEDICAL CENTER
MULTI-PURPOSE ROOM

THE TEACHING OF CLINICAL MEDICINE
Abbas Sedaghat, M.D., Professor of Medicine, University of California San Diego
Chief, General Internal Medicine and Geriatrics
San Diego VA HealthCare Center

The monthly list of Grand Rounds at UCSD and the VA Medical Center.

Many accomplished physicians do not return to Iran following the completion of their training abroad. A variety of factors may play a role in this behavior. These include the relatively poor financial returns for the efforts put into achieving their status, the restrictions and difficulties of daily living in Iran, and their concern regarding the political future of the country.

A major problem in the USA and elsewhere is the cost of medical care. This is due to the extensive and often unnecessary use of modern technology, MRI, CT scans, and multiple blood work. These tests are a major advance in medical diagnosis and therapy, but most will agree that a substantial proportion of these procedures are carried out for patient and often physician ignorance and reassurance.

Professor Peart at St. Mary's Hospital in London often quizzed his house officers regarding the need for tests ordered and carried out by them. I recall the case of a patient with Addison's Disease who had daily CBC and electrolytes done to check on his serum sodium and potassium. In these cases, because of the lack of aldosterone the sodium level is often low and the serum potassium is high. Once the diagnosis has been made, there is no longer a need for ongoing daily electrolyte measurements.

At Scripps Clinic, I would be confronted by patients with migraine who in spite of previously normal head CT/ MRI's would demand repeat testing to make doubly sure no other pathology was responsible for their symptoms.

Excessive and unnecessary testing in the majority of medical centers is a major cause of the excessively high cost of medical care. This is passed on to the patients and those who are not able to afford the absurd cost of health insurance or out of pocket expenses are bound to suffer accordingly.

I have noted with concern and sadness the lack of availability and empathy on the part of medical personnel toward their patients. Appointments are often not available within a reasonable period of time, which means that patients have to wait agonizingly for long periods of time before being seen by their physicians or other caregivers. The major systemic changes in the practice of medicine in this day and age have produced great pressures and stress on the relationship between physicians and patients, resulting in lack of availability, time, empathy, and concern. The art of medicine, which in my opinion involves the laying on of hands, seems to be vanishing with the introduction of modern computerized technology. One of the major benefits of the doctor-patient relationship is the availability of the close interaction between physician and patient. This interaction seems to be in the process of being lost. Physicians and other caregivers should be more involved with direct patient contact and show more concern and understanding toward their fellow human beings.

On retirement, it was difficult to leave the practice of medicine after so many years of success and failure. I close this tale by enclosing several letters of support from some of my colleagues at the VA Medical Center, where I spent many years of my life. I hope I have been able to train a cadre of physicians to provide essential services to patients in dire need of care, without being unduly concerned about their ability to cover the immense modern day costs of healthcare.

Awards and Accomplishments

UNIVERSITY OF LONDON

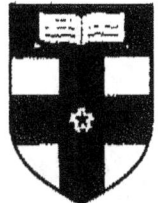

Abbas Sedaghat

of

St. Mary's Hospital Medical School

having completed the course of study approved by the University

and passed the prescribed examinations as an Internal Student

has this day been admitted by the Senate to the degrees of

BACHELOR OF MEDICINE

and

BACHELOR OF SURGERY

24 May 1964

James Henderson
Academic Registrar

QUALIFICATION TO PRACTISE MEDICINE, SURGERY AND MIDWIFERY

I, *Edward Charles Dodds Bt. M.V.*, President of the Royal College of Physicians of London, with the consent of the Fellows of the same College, have under the authority given to us by Royal Charter and Act of Parliament, granted to *Abbas Sedaghat* who has satisfied the College of his proficiency, our Licence under the said Charter to practise Physic, including therein the practice of Medicine, Surgery, and Midwifery, so long as he shall continue to obey the Statutes, Bye-Laws, and Regulations of the College relating to Licentiates, in witness whereof we have this day set our Seal and Signature Dated at the College the thirtieth day of April in the year of our Lord one thousand nine hundred and sixty four

E.C. Dodds _____ President

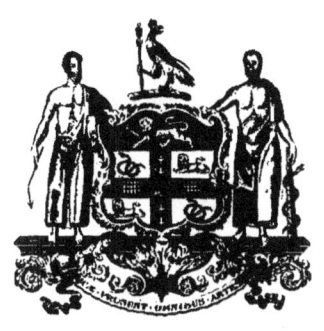

The Court of Examiners
of the
Royal College of Surgeons of England
having found

Abbas Sedaghat

to be duly qualified in the
Science and Art of Surgery
We, The Royal College of Surgeons of England
do hereby issue our Letters Testimonial, that he is qualified to practise Surgery and do hereby admit him a
Member of the College

Given under our Common Seal, this
14th day of May 1964.

Russell Brock — President.

Enrolled by _____ Secretary.

Signature of Member. Abbas Sedaghat

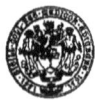  

This is to certify that

ABBAS SEDAGHAT

having satisfied the Examiners in APRIL 1970 has been duly elected to the Membership of the

Royal Colleges of Physicians of the United Kingdom

_____ President
Royal College of Physicians of Edinburgh

_____ President
_____ Visitor
Royal College of Physicians and Surgeons of Glasgow

_____ President
Royal College of Physicians of London

_____ Member

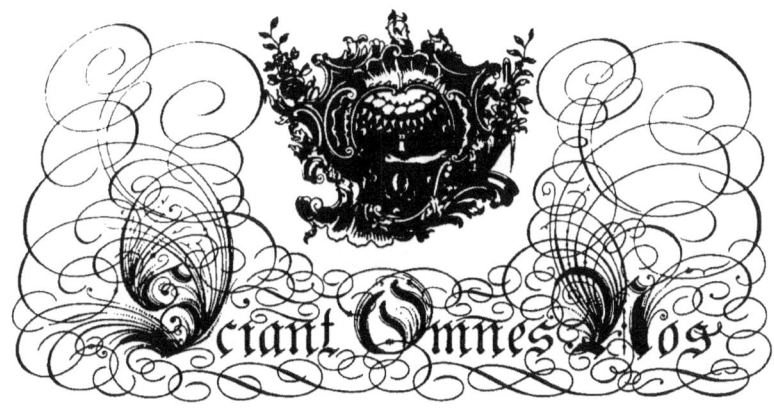

Sciant Omnes Nos

Sir Raymond Hoffenberg

Medicinæ Doctorem et Præsidentem Collegii Regalis Medicorum Londinensis, una cum consensu Sociorum ejusdem Collegii, auctoritate nobis a domino Rege et Parliamento concessa, approbasse et in Societatem nostram cooptasse doctum et probum virum

Abbas Sedaghat

In Florentissima Academia Londiniensi Medicinae Doctorem largitosque, præterea, usum et fructum omnium commoditatum, libertatum ac privilegiorum, quæ Collegio nostro auctoritate prædicta et jam concessa sunt et in futurum concedenda.

In cujus rei fidem et testimonium Sigillum nostrum commune præsentibus apponi fecimus. Datum Londini in Collegio nostro **Tricesimo** die mensis **Aprilis** Annoque Domini Millesimo noningentesimo **Octogesimo Septimo**

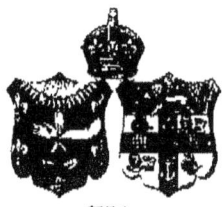

We
The President and Fellows
of
The Royal College of Physicians of London
and
We
The President and Council
of
The Royal College of Surgeons of England
have granted this

Diploma in Anæsthetics

to

Abbas Sedaghat

who has satisfied us of his proficiency in this subject.

In Witness whereof We the Presidents have hereunto set our signatures.

Dated this 25th day of July 1966

President of the Royal College of Physicians of London.   President of the Royal College of Surgeons of England.

Signature of Diplomate

UNIVERSITY OF LONDON

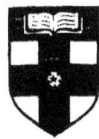

ABBAS SEDAGHAT

has this day been admitted by the Senate

as an Internal Student to the degree of

DOCTOR OF MEDICINE

20 APRIL 1977

Frank Hartley
Vice-Chancellor

DEPARTMENT OF Consumer Affairs

The Board of Medical Quality Assurance
OF THE STATE OF CALIFORNIA

This is to Certify, That **Sedaghat Abbas**, a graduate of **University of London Faculty of Medicine** having shown to the satisfaction of this Board that he possesses the qualifications required by law, and having produced a certificate entitling him to practice medicine and surgery issued by the **New York State Board for Medicine** on the **10th** day of **October**, 19**72**, which complies with the requirements of the Business and Professions Code of the State of California, relating to the practice of medicine and surgery, is hereby granted a

RECIPROCITY

Physician's and Surgeon's Certificate

IN THIS STATE

In Testimony Whereof, THE BOARD OF MEDICAL QUALITY ASSURANCE of the STATE OF CALIFORNIA has issued this CERTIFICATE and caused the same to be signed by its PRESIDENT and SECRETARY-TREASURER and its SEAL to be hereto affixed this **29th** day of **May**, A.D. 19**79**

The Board of Medical Quality Assurance
OF THE STATE OF CALIFORNIA

President

No. C **38672**

THE AMERICAN BOARD OF INTERNAL MEDICINE

INCORPORATED 1936

ORGANIZED
THROUGH THE CO-OPERATION OF THE
AMERICAN COLLEGE OF PHYSICIANS
AND THE SECTION ON THE PRACTICE OF MEDICINE OF THE
AMERICAN MEDICAL ASSOCIATION

ATTESTS THAT

Abbas Sedaghat

HAS MET THE REQUIREMENTS OF THIS BOARD AND IS HEREBY DESIGNATED A
DIPLOMATE CERTIFIED TO PRACTICE THE SPECIALTY OF

INTERNAL MEDICINE

MEMBER 40888

DATE JUNE 21, 1972

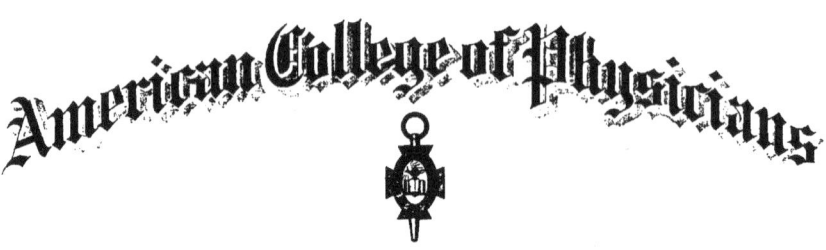

American College of Physicians

Be it known to all to whom these letters may come that

Abbas Sedaghat

has been elected a

Fellow of the American College of Physicians

In witness whereof the Seal of the College and the signatures of the proper officers are affixed.

Given in the City of Philadelphia, this tenth *day of* November *in the year 1979.*

Richard W. Vilter
President

Julius E. Scott
Secretary General

Letters of Recommendation

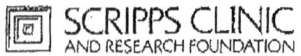 **SCRIPPS CLINIC AND RESEARCH FOUNDATION**

SCRIPPS CLINIC MEDICAL GROUP, INC.
10666 NORTH TORREY PINES ROAD
LA JOLLA, CALIFORNIA 92037
619 455-9100

Donald J. Dalessio, M.D.
Senior Consultant
Division of Neurology
Chairman
Department of Medicine

April 29, 1988

TO WHOM IT MAY CONCERN:

Dr. A. Sedaghat has been a member of the Department of Medicine (Division of General Internal Medicine) here at the Scripps Clinic and Research Foundation since 1979.

He has had excellent training in medicine both in this country and in Britain. He has achieved selection to the fellowship of the American College of Physicians as well as the Royal College of Physicians of Great Britain.

Dr. Sedaghat is an excellent Internist who has worked hard and diligently at this institution over the years. His Grand Rounds presentations won him first prize in 1984 and second prize in 1986. He has taken an active part in the training of Physicians in our Residency program for several years.

He is an invaluable member of our medical group and we look forward to having him back with us soon.

Sincerely,

D. Dalessio, M.D.

DD/csl

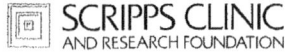

SCRIPPS CLINIC MEDICAL GROUP, INC.
10666 NORTH TORREY PINES ROAD
LA JOLLA, CALIFORNIA 92037
619 455-9100

Anthony P. Moore, M.D.
Head
Division of General Internal Medicine

November 27, 1988

To Whom It May Concern:

Dr. Abbas Sedaghat has been a member of the Division of General Internal Medicine at Scripps Clinic since 1979. He came with impeccable credentials having had superb training in the United Kingdom of Great Britain and in the United States of America.

Dr. Sedaghat has had extensive research experience in the field of lipid metabolism and is the Director of the Lipid Disorders Clinic at this institution. He is an astute clinician with many diagnostic coups to his credit. He and I shared first prize in Grand Rounds in 1984 for our presentation of several fascinating diagnostic problems. His clinical ability is respected and lauded by his peers and the house staff at this institution and at the University of California in San Diego School of Medicine where he is Associate Clinical Professor of Medicine.

Dr. Sedaghat has a large following of patients who are dedicated to him because of his humane concern for their problems and his unflagging efforts to resolve them. He is personable, kind, considerate and utterly reliable.

It has been a pleasure to have had Dr. Sedaghat as a friend and colleague over the years. His departure will be a blow to Scripps Clinic where he will be sorely missed.

Sincerely,

Anthony P. Moore, M.D.
Head, Division of General Internal Medicine

UNIVERSITY OF CALIFORNIA, SAN DIEGO UCSD

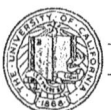

BERKELEY · DAVIS · IRVINE · LOS ANGELES · RIVERSIDE · SAN DIEGO · SAN FRANCISCO   SANTA BARBARA · SANTA CRUZ

OFFICE OF THE DEAN, 0602
SCHOOL OF MEDICINE

9500 GILMAN DRIVE
LA JOLLA, CALIFORNIA 92093-0602

April 19, 1991

Abbas Sedaghat, M.D.
VA Medical Center
V-111

Dear Dr. Sedaghat:

I am pleased to offer you an appointment as Clinical Professor, Step I, in the Department of Medicine as a member of the faculty of the School of Medicine at the University of California, San Diego, retroactive to January 1, 1991 through June 30, 1993. This offer is made concurrent with your appointment at the Veterans Administration Hospital as Grade 15, Step 10 level, 8/8 time.

Faculty who are employed by the VA and who are involved in patient care activities in University facilities may participate in the "Z" component of the Plan. Any questions you have about the application of this plan to your personal situation should be directed to your department chair.

An initial appointment in the salaried Clinical series is normally for the period of review, in your case three years, subject to the availability of funds. Your appointment represents an important phase in the joint endeavor of the UCSD School of Medicine and the Veterans Administration Hospital to provide the best in medical care.

Please contact your department regarding application procedures for Medical Staff privileges.

Your signature is not required on the Status Change Form which will implement this action; however, you will need to sign the MSCCP Statement of Agreement * and return it in the enclosed envelope to signify your official acceptance. Upon receipt of the signed form we will process the necessary papers to implement the appointment.

Sincerely,

Paul J. Friedman, M.D.
Dean for Academic Affairs

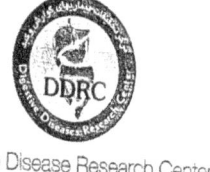 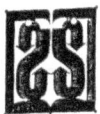

Digestive Disease Research Center
Tehran University of Medical Sciences

Date: ....
Ref: ....

R. Malekzadeh M.D.
Professor of Medicine & Gastroenterology
Director, Digestive Disease Research Center
Tehran University of Medical Sciences
Kargar Shomali Ave, Shariati Hospital,
14114 Tehran / Iran
Tel: +98 – 21 – 8012992
Fax: +98 – 21 – 2253635
E-mail: malek@iams.ac.ir

5th May 2001

Dear Dr. Sedaghat

I and my colleagues would like to express our gratitude for your kind cooperation in the educational and training activities of our students, residents and fellows at the Digestive Disease Research Center, Tehran University of Medical Sciences. Your patient and enthusiastic manner in teaching at our department will be remembered by all. We wish you the best and are looking forward to your future collaboration with our department.

Best Regards
R. Malekzadeh

UNIVERSITY OF CALIFORNIA, SAN DIEGO   UCSD

BERKELEY · DAVIS · IRVIINE · LOS ANGELES · RIVERSIDE · SAN DIEGO · SAN FRANCISCO 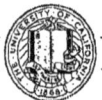 SANTA BARBARA· SANTA CRUZ

SIMERJOT K. JASSAL, M.D.
ASSISTANT CLINICAL PROFESSOR
DEPARTMENT OF INTERNAL MEDICINE
SCHOOL OF MEDICINE
VA SAN DIEGO HEALTHCARE SYSTEM

3350 LA JOLLA VILLAGE DRIVE
DIVISION OF GIM/G, MC 9111N
SAN DIEGO, CALIFORNIA 92161
(858) 552-8585 x2881
E-mail: sjassal@ucsd.edu

July 28, 2006

To Whom It May Concern:

It is my pleasure to write this letter of recommendation on behalf of Dr. Abbas Sedaghat. He is an outstanding clinician, teacher and mentor and will undoubtedly be a welcome addition to your institution.

I have had the opportunity to work with Dr. Sedaghat during the past four years. As a staff physician in the section of General Internal Medicine and Geriatrics at the VA San Diego Healthcare System, Dr. Sedaghat has been my supervisor and our section chief. Throughout this time, I have found him to be a capable leader and staunch advocate for the members of our section. Under his leadership, our section has grown and added physicians of outstanding caliber. He has mentored and supported me in all of my professional endeavors in the research and educational realms, allowing me to advance my career as a clinician-educator. Throughout the course of his career here at UCSD, Dr. Sedaghat has won numerous teaching awards from the medical students who laud him as a master clinician and an expert in teaching physical exam skills—an area that is quickly becoming a lost art. I strive to one day become expert teacher that Dr. Sedaghat is. His retirement will be a loss to our institution, our section and our residents and students.

It is with great enthusiasm that I endorse the application of Dr. Abbas Sedaghat to your healthcare system. If I can be of any further assistance or provide you with any additional information, please do not hesitate to contact me.

Sincerely,

Simerjot K. Jassal, M.D.
Assistant Clinical Professor
Associate Program Director
Residency Training Program
Department of Internal Medicine
UCSD School of Medicine

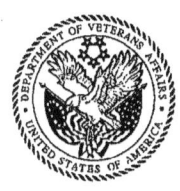

ADRIAN W. DOLLARHIDE, MD
DEPARTMENT OF VETERANS AFFAIRS
VA San Diego Healthcare System
Division of General Internal Medicine
Mail Code 111-N
San Diego CA 92161
Telephone: (858)552-7475

July 30, 2006

To Whom It May Concern,

I have had the distinct pleasure over the past seven years of considering Dr. Abbas Sedaghat an esteemed colleague, and I am flattered by his request to offer my support in a letter of recommendation. Quite simply put, Dr. Sedaghat has a wealth of clinical experience and diagnostic talent. He is widely known for his mastery of the art of the physical examination, and has passed on these skills to hundreds of fortunate medical students and residents throughout his years at the UCSD School of Medicine. For his efforts, Dr. Sedaghat has been awarded numerous Outstanding Teacher of the Year awards, reflecting both his skill and leadership.

Dr. Sedaghat's knowledge base and ability to ascertain the correct clinical diagnosis have made him *the* physician to whom all students, residents and staff colleagues alike naturally gravitate toward when presented with a particularly challenging or baffling case. His diagnostic acumen seems only paralleled by his clinical and therapeutic skills, and the respect and trust he elicits from the patients he treats. He is truly the physicians' physician, leading by example and tirelessly supporting the efforts and aspirations of those fortunate enough to be around him.

As the leader of the Section of General Internal Medicine at the VA San Diego, he has hand-crafted and overseen the phenomenal growth and expansion of the most clinically productive section in our hospital. He has shepherded this growth through his deliberate sense of pride, professionalism, and devotion to delivering the absolute best in medical care available. I am very pleased to offer my most enthusiastic support for Dr. Sedaghat in his future career. Please feel free to contact me personally if I can be of any further assistance.

Sincerely,

Adrian W. Dollarhide, MD
Associate Clinical Professor of Medicine
University of California, San Diego

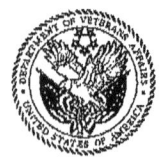

COLIN M. THOMAS MD, MPH
DEPARTMENT OF VETERANS AFFAIRS
VA San Diego Healthcare System
Division of General Internal Medicine and Geriatrics
Associate Clinical Professor of Medicine
UCSD School of Medicine
Mail Code 111-N
San Diego CA 92161
Telephone: (858)552-8585 x 2811

20 July 2006

To whom it may concern:

I have worked closely with Dr. Abbas Sedaghat over the past eleven years. His patient care is excellent in both the primary care and urgent care settings. He takes a leadership role in the clinic. His teaching awards are so numerous that he withdrew his name from consideration to give others a chance. He is a staunch advocate for quality patient care and for his colleagues' ability to practice quality medicine. I am confident he will be an asset to your institution and I recommend him enthusiastically. Please feel free to contact me if you require further information.

Colin M. Thomas MD, MPH

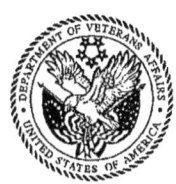

DEPARTMENT OF VETERANS AFFAIRS
San Diego Healthcare System
3350 La Jolla Village Drive
San Diego CA 92161

August 1, 2006

To Whom It May Concern:

I would like to offer my strongest recommendation for Dr. Abbas Sedaghat. I had the pleasure of working under his leadership as the Section Chief of General Internal Medicine/Geriatrics here at the San Diego VA Medical Center. He served in the capacity of section chief for almost 16 years. During those 16 years, he received numerous letters of commendation and teaching awards, both from the medical students as well as the internal medicine housestaff. He has proven himself to be one of the best teachers this hospital has ever produced, and one of the best teachers I have ever had in my career.

Along with being an academic powerhouse, Dr. Sedaghat is also a very caring physician. He has always shown compassion toward his patients, ensuring they receive all the care needed by them. Simply put, he is the physician's physician. I would not hesistate to be one of his patients nor send any of my family members to him.

I have told Dr. Sedaghat before that if I could be half as good as he is, I would have considered myself to have had a successful career. Dr. Sedaghat will be one of the greatest assets you will have at your institution. It is without any reservations that I offer my highest recommendation for Dr. Sedaghat. If any questions, please feel free to call me anytime at (858) 552-8585 x 2811. Thank you.

Sincerely,

Tuan Dang, MD

UNIVERSITY OF CALIFORNIA, SAN DIEGO 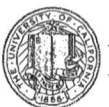 UCSD

BERKELEY • DAVIS • IRVINE • LOS ANGELES • MERCED • RIVERSIDE • SAN DIEGO • SAN FRANCISCO   SANTA BARBARA • SANTA CRUZ

DEPARTMENT OF MEDICINE
SCHOOL OF MEDICINE

VETERANS AFFAIRS MEDICAL CENTER
3350 LA JOLLA VILLAGE DRIVE
SAN DIEGO, CALIFORNIA 92161

July 21, 2006

To Whom It May Concern:

I am writing this letter to communicate my thoughts about Dr. Abbas Sedaghat.

I met Dr. Sedaghat when I moved to San Diego in 1998 and began working at the VA Hospital there as an internist. At that time and for many years thereafter, Dr. Sedaghat was Section Chief of Internal Medicine. Throughout the period that I worked with him, I had the distinct pleasure of seeing him run a large and growing Internal Medicine Staff. I also saw another side of his talent – his rare and distinguished ability to teach and mentor.

In the almost ten years that I have known Abbas, I can say that his internal medicine skills are superb. He makes very reasonable use of ancillary diagnostic tools, but he relies very much on the physical examination. And almost always he has the diagnosis from his examination alone! That is something modern medicine is losing, yet he has a true gift for it.

As my supervisor, Dr. Sedaghat always provided the kind of mentorship that anyone would wish for. His leadership steered me in directions that laid critical foundations for my own career pathway, and I would venture to say that everyone in our Internal Medicine Section would state the same.

In summary, I can recommend Dr. Abbas Sedaghat to you with the very highest level of enthusiasm. You can be confident he will be the strongest of assets to your team.

Sincerely,

Mark T. Gabuzda, MD
Veterans Affairs Medical Center
Associate Professor of Medicine
University of San Diego, California

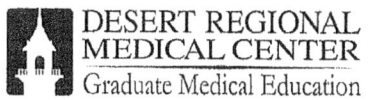

KATRINA PLATT, DO, FACOI
RESIDENCY PROGRAM DIRECTOR, INTERNAL MEDICINE

April 16, 2018

RE: Dr. Abbas Sedaghat

To Whom It May Concern,

I would like to write to you with my strong recommendation for you to consider Dr. Abbas Sedaghat for employment with your practice or facility. He came to my residency at Desert Regional Medical Center as a Locum when we were in need for attending supervision in the Internal Medicine Resident Continuity Clinic. Dr. Sedaghat is a true diagnostician. He utilizes the fundamental techniques of medicine to diagnose and treat. He appreciated the patient as a whole which I appreciate as an Osteopathic Physician. The residents he supervises praise him for the time he takes to listen and teach.

He has gone above and beyond what is expected for his employment and has volunteered to run morning report with the residents on a weekly basis. In between patients, I see him studying Harrison's chapters to keep up to date with the residents. He has a very kind demeanor and is well liked by the staff, residents, and patients. He will definitely be an asset wherever he goes and he will be missed.

If you have any questions please feel free to contact me directly and I would be happy to discuss further.

Sincerely,

Katrina Platt, DO

1100 N. PALM CANYON DRIVE, SUITE 109 | PALM SPRINGS, CA 92262
T: 760-992-7152 | F: 760-327-3846

Date: Thursday, October 6, 2005

Subject: General Internal Medicine - Geriatrics Section

After 15 years of service as head of the General Internal Medicine / Geriatrics Section, Dr. Abbas Sedaghat is stepping down to focus on development and implementation of strategies to enhance faculty educational efforts.

Under Dr. Sedaghat's leadership, the General Internal Medicine / Geriatrics Section has grown dramatically and has achieved recognition for outstanding educational strength. Personally, Dr. Sedaghat has been recognized for his outstanding educational abilities through receipt of many School of Medicine teaching awards. Utilizing his talents for medical instruction, Dr. Sedaghat will focus on efforts to improve teaching of both medical students and house officers.

The Medicine Service and SD VA Healthcare System are grateful to Dr. Sedaghat for his years of service, and enthusiastically anticipate his future contributions to medical education.

Roger Spragg, MD
Chief, Medicine Service
San Diego VA Healthcare System

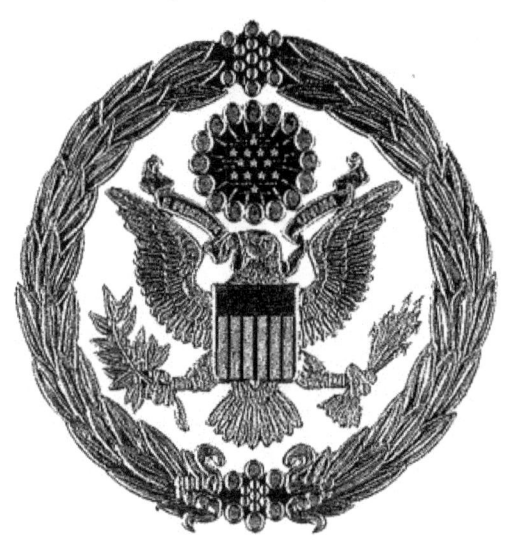

Certificate of Retirement

Honoring

Abbas Sedaghat, MD

in recognition of your retirement from the
Department of Veterans Affairs following *16* years
of dedicated service to the
Government of the United States of America.

Gary J. Rossio, CHE
Director

www.ingramcontent.com/pod-product-compliance
Lightning Source LLC
Chambersburg PA
CBHW071117160426
43196CB00013B/2596